PATTERNS OF HOSPITAL OWNERSHIP
AND CONTROL

PATTERNS

of Hospital Ownership and Control

by JAMES A. HAMILTON, PROFESSOR AND DIRECTOR
PROGRAM IN HOSPITAL ADMINISTRATION, UNIVERSITY OF MINNESOTA

with the assistance of
R. Bruce Butters, M.H.A., *and* Elbert E. Gilbertson, M.H.A.

UNIVERSITY OF MINNESOTA PRESS Minneapolis

Preface

In order that both beginning and experienced students of hospital administration might advance their understanding of the nearly seven thousand independent units of hospital service in the United States, this study was undertaken. It seemed necessary for securing such understanding to arrange the mass of units in a series of clearly defined patterns, to describe the characteristics of each pattern, and to indicate the relationship of each to the whole. This arrangement of *producing* units of service, which was originally intended to be merely a single chapter of a textbook, has gradually become a sizable volume in itself, the result of a long-term project of collecting and processing information.

Most of the data already existed in more or less gross form; yet apparently no previous attempt had been made to arrange and classify this information for study or to interpret its significance as a whole. Once the basic outline had been determined and considerable amounts of material accumulated, additional data had to be collected from various sources to ascertain the meaning of the newer patterns.

Much of the effort that gave the material its final form represents a year's work by each of two recent graduates of the Program in Hospital Administration at the University of Minnesota. The late R. Bruce Butters broke the barriers to assemble the source materials, develop the approach and general outline, and perform the initial writing. Elbert E. Gilbertson struggled with rearrangement, included newer patterns, updated most of the material, and completed the bulk of the writing. Appreciation is given to Ernest Holman and Lawrence Hill for their review of the galley proofs.

The first year's work was financed by the W. K. Kellogg Foundation and the later years by James A. Hamilton Associates.

It was surprising to discover how little writing had been done about the patterns within the broader classifications — for example, a specific church-owned and/or -operated hospital group. It is our hope that administrators of some of these hospitals, stimulated by this effort, will not concentrate in the future solely on collecting data about their individual hospital but will do so about their entire group, unfold in greater detail the group's operation, and publish their findings.

In the meantime, this volume may help in developing the *conceptual skill* of students preparing for careers in this service of increasing significance in modern society.

JAMES A. HAMILTON

June, 1961

Table of Contents

List of Figures

PATTERNS OF HOSPITAL OWNERSHIP
AND CONTROL

Little do ye know your own blessedness . . .

ROBERT LOUIS STEVENSON

Independence? That's middle-class blasphemy. We are all dependent on one another, every soul of us on earth.

GEORGE BERNARD SHAW

Introduction

THE primary purpose of this study and report is to provide students in hospital administration with a concept of the hospital industry and the different organizations which make hospital care possible in the United States.

Most of the discussion is devoted to the various individual patterns of hospital ownership and control, and to describing briefly each pattern's organizational structure and governing authority, history, significance, finances, educational activities, administration, medical staff, groups or associations within the pattern, and future trends. Length of description varies among the patterns, not as an indication of relative importance, but according to the amount of information available for each pattern.

No attempt has been made to completely exhaust the hospital field. However, the study does include a description of most of the more significant and better known ownership and control patterns. It also describes some patterns under which relatively few hospitals are operated but whose characteristics are unique.

Osteopathic hospitals do not fit the definition of "hospital" used in this study nor the statistical collection of the American Hospital Association. As a result, they are excluded from consideration in Parts I and II. Also, they do not represent a separate and distinct ownership and control pattern, but differ in the composition of their medical staffs. Nevertheless, they are included in an addendum for two reasons. First, there are a relatively large number of these institutions in the United States and they have a significant effect on the total hospital picture in this country. Second, if the present medical and osteopathic professions ever merge, as the medical and homeopathic professions did approximately fifty years ago, osteopathic hospitals will then be absorbed and included in the ownership and control patterns and statistics presented in the other parts of the study.

3

Patterns of Hospital Ownership and Control

Although the greatest part of the statistical information was taken from the 1957 Guide Issue of *Hospitals*, the official publication of the American Hospital Association, many other organizations also contributed data on specific patterns. While most of the statistics pertain to the year 1956, some of the patterns — particularly those covering federal hospitals — have been updated to 1957 or 1958. However, the fact that figures from different years have been used does not appear to be a serious shortcoming for the purposes of this study. The statistical information is presented merely to illustrate the size of the various patterns and their significance in relation to each other and to the total hospital industry. Neither their size nor their relative significance changes greatly from year to year.

Moreover, from a statistical standpoint, much desired data could not be secured at this time and it was necessary to make estimates. These estimations were determined as carefully and accurately as possible, and they have been checked and reviewed by the organizations which supplied information on individual patterns. Nevertheless, the reader is warned against placing complete reliance on the exactness of all the figures presented. They should be used as general guides only.

Although comparison of the various patterns is invited and encouraged, the reader is cautioned also against interpreting these comparisons too freely in order to applaud one pattern or condemn another. This is especially true of the statistical *averages* that have been used. For example, a much higher operating cost per patient day in one pattern as compared with another may be justified when all factors have been considered and may not be attributable to inefficient management or subject to some other equally condemning interpretation.

Thus, while the study is admittedly imperfect and limited, it is believed that it will accomplish its major purpose of providing beginning students in the field with a concept of the hospital industry and the different existing patterns of hospital ownership and control. It is expected also that the study will be a source of reference for, and add to the knowledge of, veteran personnel in hospitals. Finally, it is hoped that this imperfect beginning will stimulate others to pursue additional investigations in this area in the future.

THE HOSPITAL INDUSTRY

What is a hospital? Perhaps it is well to pose and answer this question at the very beginning; first, because the entire study is devoted to a discussion of such institutions; second, because the meaning of the word has changed considerably over the centuries. Moreover, it is well to recognize that, even today, many different definitions persist.

Obsolete Definitions. The term "hospital" has its derivation in the

4

Latin words *hospes*, meaning a stranger or guest, and *hospitalis*, relating to a guest. The word has been applied to many different types of institutions through the years. At various intervals, for example, a "hospital" has been defined as (1) a place for the shelter or entertainment of travelers and strangers; (2) a charitable institution for the refuge, maintenance, or education of needy, aged, infirm, or young persons; (3) a university hall; (4) a place of lodging, such as an inn or private mansion.

Current Definitions. Our present knowledge of the medical and related sciences is far beyond the capacity of a single individual to absorb and master, and has necessarily been dispersed into many different specialties and technologies. However, in the conservation of human health, the sum of such knowledge must be brought together and the various specialties and technologies coordinated. The hospital of today is recognized as this converging point.

As a result, any differences that exist among the current definitions of the term "hospital" are largely a matter of interpretation. Most hospital authorities or agencies concerned with gathering hospital statistics would basically agree with the 1956 edition of *Webster's New Collegiate Dictionary* that a hospital is "an institution in which patients or injured persons are given medical or surgical care." However, some authorities and agencies interpret this definition freely and consider almost all institutions rendering care to the sick to be hospitals. Others are more restrictive in their interpretation and regard as hospitals only those institutions meeting certain requirements over and above those already imposed by the dictionary definition.

Among the latter are the various state governments, each of which has a set of requirements that must be satisfied before an institution in its domain can be licensed as a hospital. In Minnesota, for example, a hospital is defined as "an institution adequately and properly staffed and equipped; providing services, facilities and beds for the reception and care for a continuous period longer than 12 hours, for one or more non-related persons requiring diagnosis, treatment or care for illness, injury or pregnancy; and regularly making available clinical laboratory services, diagnostic X-ray services, and treatment facilities for (a) surgery or (b) obstetrical care or (c) other definitive medical treatment of similar extent."

The American Hospital Association has even tighter restrictions. To be accepted for listing in the directory of hospitals published annually by this association, an institution must comply with the following requirements:

1. The hospital shall have at least six beds for the care of patients who

are nonrelated, who are sick and who stay on the average in excess of 24 hours per admission.

2. The hospital shall be licensed in those states and provinces having licensing laws.

3. Only doctors of medicine or doctors of osteopathy shall practice in hospitals listed by the American Hospital Association. (This requirement is not intended to eliminate dental and similar services from the hospital. Patients admitted for such services, however, must have an admission history and a physical examination done by a physician on the staff of the hospital, and a physician on the staff of the hospital shall be responsible for the patient's medical care throughout his stay.)

4. Duly authorized bylaws for the medical staff shall be adopted by the hospital.

5. The hospital shall submit evidence of regular care of the patient by the attending physician and of general supervision of the clinical work by doctors of medicine.

6. Records of clinical work shall be maintained by the hospital on all patients and shall be available for reference.

7. Registered nurse supervision and such other nursing service as is necessary to provide patient care around the clock shall be available at the hospital.

8. The hospital shall offer services more intensive than those required merely for room, board, personal services, and general nursing care.

9. Minimal surgical or obstetrical facilities, including operating or delivery room, or relatively complete diagnostic facilities and treatment facilities for medical patients, shall be available at the hospital.

10. Diagnostic X-ray services shall be regularly and conveniently available.

11. Clinical laboratory services shall be regularly and conveniently available.

The American Hospital Association's directory is by far the best source of hospital data available and most of the statistical information in the following chapters was taken from it. For this reason, the requirements for listing in the directory constitute the definition of "hospital" that will be used in this study.

As a result, the study does not discuss institutions which fail to meet these qualifications such as nursing homes, clinics, and diagnostic and treatment centers. Acceptance of these requirements as a definition of "hospital" does not exclude institutions having one or more doctors of osteopathy on their staffs from consideration in Parts I and II of the study. As previously indicated, however, osteopathic hospitals are discussed in an addendum because of the relatively large number of such institutions and because of the possibility that some day the osteopathic and the medical professions will merge, with the consequent absorption of osteopathic hospitals into other patterns of hospital ownership and control.

The Nation's Hospitals. Hospitals in the United States today are rapidly becoming community health centers providing ever-broadening programs of improved health services and facilities.

While many countries have developed single government plans for hospital care, it will become increasingly apparent to the reader, as he goes through this study, that the demands made on the hospital industry in the United States are so large and complex that it would have been and will continue to be impossible for any individual or governmental agency to develop a single pattern or plan.

In little more than a century of dramatic and spectacular progress in health care programs, our present voluntary hospital system is a tribute to the loyal support and good will of the American people. The ability of the American people to adequately meet and solve well their future health care needs will depend primarily on a continued extension of a favorable atmosphere for the application of the principle of freedom of enterprise. Progress in hospital care can flourish best when it is unhampered and unrestrained by bureaucratic and political considerations and when the climate countenances no barriers to the exercise of initiative, ingenuity, and resourcefulness. Of course the voluntary hospital groups must maintain cooperative relationships with federal, state, and local governing bodies, as they, too, seek to fulfill their respective obligations to the citizenry through government-sponsored health care programs and hospital facilities.

The first hospital census was taken in this country in 1873. It revealed only 178 units with a combined capacity of approximately 35,000 beds, one third of which were reserved for the mentally ill. Since that time, the number of hospitals has multiplied thirty-nine times and the number of beds nearly forty-six times.

Hospital beds have increased at a faster rate than the nation's population. In the early 1900s there were less than 5 hospital beds per thousand population. By 1956, the ratio had jumped to 9.6 beds per thousand.

There has been a significant rise in the utilization of hospitals in recent years. On the average day in 1956 more than 1,350,000 people — slightly less than 1 per cent of our total population — were hospitalized, a 19 per cent increase over 1946 (see Table 1).

The number of admissions rose 41 per cent in the same period. During 1956 a hospital admission was recorded every one and a half seconds. In addition, a live baby was delivered in a hospital every nine seconds in that year.

7

Patterns of Hospital Ownership and Control

Table 1. Growth of Hospitals in the Continental United States from 1946 to 1956

	1946	1956	% of Increase
Number of hospitals	6,125	6,966	14
Number of beds	1,435,778	1,607,692	12
Average daily census	1,141,864	1,355,792	19
Annual admissions	15,674,602	22,089,719	41
Number of paid personnel	829,571*	1,374,704	66
Assets	$5,300,000,000†	$13,035,068,000	146†
Annual expenses	$1,963,355,000	$ 6,016,859,000	206
Annual payroll expenses	$1,102,772,000	$ 3,948,937,000	258

* Includes full-time equivalents of part-time personnel but excludes residents, interns, and students.

† Estimated.

Nearly 500 million patient days of care were rendered by our hospitals in 1956, a figure equal to the total average life span of 20,000 persons.

In the same year, the total assets of the hospitals in this country were evaluated at more than $13 billion, an investment of $78 for every American and estimated to be just under 1 per cent of the nation's total wealth. Hospital assets multiplied almost one and a half times in the period from 1946 to 1956. Most of this increase was in new construction stimulated after World War II by passage of the federal Hospital Survey and Construction Act. Commonly referred to as the Hill-Burton Act, it provides federal funds, on a matching basis, for the construction of new hospital facilities.

United States hospitals expended over $6 billion in 1956, or roughly $11,500 every minute. The tremendous increase in total expenditures from 1946 to 1956 — more than 200 per cent — was primarily due to the even more significant rise in payroll expenses in the same period. The latter resulted from the advent of the forty-hour work week and the payment of higher salaries as well as the addition of personnel to provide the ever-expanding services hospital patients deserve and demand. Currently, salaries and wages account for almost two thirds of the total hospital expense dollar.

The gigantic rise in both total and payroll expenditures in the 1946–1956 interval purchased new drugs, equipment, and personnel, which, together with the very rapid advances made in the medical sciences, permitted hospitals to render a higher quality of patient care. This was reflected in the decrease in the average length of patient stay in non-federal short-term general and special hospitals from 9.1 days in 1946 to 7.7 days in 1956.

Nearly 1,400,000 persons — about 2 per cent of the nation's total civilian labor force — were employed in our hospitals in 1956. The 66 per cent increase in personnel in the period from 1946 to 1956 corresponded with a similar rise in the number of employees per patient. In 1946, all hospitals averaged 73 employees for every 100 patients. Eleven years later, there were 101 employees for the same number of patients.

Hospitals as an Industry. The general public rarely has an opportunity to observe the entire operation of a hospital. Even patients and visitors normally are confined to a few hospital areas and are directly served by a small proportion of the total personnel. As a result, it is not too surprising that most people find it difficult to think of hospitals as complex enterprises of considerable size. The majority of persons would be amazed to learn, for example, that in many communities, perhaps their own, the local hospital is the town's biggest employer and operates the largest hotel, laundry, pharmacy, and restaurant. They would be even more surprised to learn that, collectively, hospitals make up one of the country's largest industries and are a vital cog in the nation's economic structure.

True, most hospitals are operated on a nonprofit basis and have motives and incentives different from other business enterprises. Patient service and patient comfort, rather than "profit," are the prime considerations of a hospital. As Raymond P. Sloan so aptly stated in his book, *This Hospital Business of Ours*: "From the standpoint of sound business, a hospital may be thoroughly justified in voting against expending certain sums on a specific piece of equipment. From the standpoint of a human life, it cannot refuse. Business judgment must be tempered at all times with a keen sense of social obligation. The end product is public health, not financial gain."

Nevertheless, the fact that hospitals are a business — a big business — is indisputable. For example, the hospitals in this country have more employees than the automobile, or steel, or telecommunications industries; greater total assets than the tobacco manufacturing or mining industries; higher total annual expenses than the nation's electric light and power companies, the gas utility and pipeline industry. Total annual hospital payroll expenditures are triple those of the hotel and amusement industries.

The frequently quoted statement that "hospitals are the fifth largest industry in the United States" is misleading. It is virtually impossible to make such an over-all determination with any degree of accuracy because of the lack of comparative statistical information and the differing opinions as to what constitutes an "industry." However, whether hospitals rank fifth, or fifteenth, or fiftieth among the nation's industries is relatively unimportant. Their primary significance lies in the services and patient care they help provide, not in the impact they have on the country's economy.

THE CLASSIFICATION OF HOSPITALS

Hospitals in the United States may be classified or grouped in a number of different ways, more commonly by (1) type of medical service; (2) adult bed capacity; (3) average length of patient stay; (4) geographic location; (5) ownership and control.

Type of Medical Service. The hospitals in the United States may be grossly separated by the types of medical service they render into "general" and "special" hospitals. A general hospital is one which provides treatment for a variety of medical conditions. A special hospital, on the other hand, normally limits its services to patients suffering from a specific illness or disease, such as tuberculosis, or to a particular medical specialty, such as orthopedics or pediatrics.

The more common types of special hospitals are listed in Table 2, which also illustrates the abundance of general hospitals and the extent to which they overshadow the hospital scene. Even though they contain less than one half of the total hospital beds, these general institutions make up nearly four fifths of all the nation's hospitals, admit over 95 per cent of all hospital patients, and account for more than two thirds of all hospital assets, total expenses, payroll expenses, and personnel. Most general hospitals have a relatively short average patient stay of between five and ten days. This is reflected in Table 2 by their large volume of admissions in comparison with their proportionately small number of beds.

Of particular importance among the specialized institutions are the psychiatric or mental hospitals. Although they represent less than one twelfth of all hospitals in this country and an even smaller proportion of the total hospital admissions, they contain almost 50 per cent of all hospital beds. In addition, over one half of all hospital patients on the average day are in psychiatric institutions.

Persons suffering from mental illness normally require extensive treatment and, if admitted or committed to an institution, are usually hospitalized for extremely long periods. As it is virtually impossible for most people to finance such treatment and hospitalization on a private basis, the care of the mentally ill has traditionally been a primary responsibility of the various state governments. At present approximately nine out of every ten beds in psychiatric hospitals are contained in state-owned institutions.

A fairly recent development is the addition of psychiatric units to some of the larger general hospitals. Patients entering such facilities avoid the stigma of having been admitted or committed to an "insane

Table 2. Comparative Analysis of Continental United States Hospitals, Classified by Type of Medical Service, for 1956

Type of Medical Service	No. of Hospitals	No. of Beds	Av. Daily Census†	Annual Admissions†	No. of Paid Personnel†	Assets†	Annual Expenses†	Annual Pay-roll Expenses†
General*	5,506	696,978	515,273	21,027,210	973,496	$ 8,834,023,000	$4,228,564,000	$2,737,124,000
Psychiatric	569	762,294	722,001	390,742	244,510	2,685,188,000	1,094,869,000	755,764,000
Tuberculosis	342	76,380	61,731	97,381	56,077	602,767,000	256,386,000	173,188,000
Maternity	72	3,108	1,904	94,616				
Eye, ear, nose, and throat	48	2,154	1,226	114,808				
Children's	55	6,680	4,681	199,094				
Orthopedic	81	6,567	4,806	35,043				
Contagious disease	12	1,397	475	9,546				
Chronic and convalescent.	207	41,168	35,060	59,111				
All other	74	10,966	8,635	62,168	100,621‡	913,090,000‡	437,040,000‡	282,911,000‡
Total	6,966	1,607,692	1,355,792	22,089,719	1,374,704	$13,035,068,000	$6,016,859,000	$3,948,937,000

* Includes hospital departments of institutions such as prisons, reformatories, etc.
† Estimated.
‡ Combined for the preceding seven types of medical service.

11

asylum" and are consequently encouraged to seek early diagnosis and treatment which may prevent a long period of custodial care at some future date. However, although an increasing number of general hospitals are adding psychiatric units, state-owned mental institutions will continue to dominate the psychiatric hospital and bed picture for many years.

Also of significance among the special hospitals are those which limit their services to the care and treatment of tuberculosis patients. In the past several decades, tuberculosis has slowly but steadily diminished in its importance as a common disease, particularly in the United States, and is gradually being eradicated through the use of new drugs, diagnostic procedures, and surgical techniques. As a result, the number of tuberculosis hospitals and tuberculosis beds has decreased considerably in recent years. Nevertheless, the tuberculosis institutions currently in operation represent about one twentieth of all hospitals in this country and account for between 4 and 5 per cent of all hospital assets, expenses, and personnel.

Other types of special hospitals, with the exception of the chronic and convalescent institutions, have significantly declined in number in the past decade and may be expected to decline even further in the future. This is probably due to the feeling of most hospital and medical authorities that specialized institutions, unless they are sufficiently large, are neither medically nor economically sound, because they duplicate costly services already present in general hospitals.

Adult Bed Capacity. A hospital's "size" is most commonly measured by the number of adult beds it contains. Occasionally, it is meaningful to classify or group hospitals in the United States according to adult bed capacity as shown in Table 3.

From Table 3, it is evident that we are essentially a nation of small

Table 3. Census and Admissions Data for Continental United States Hospitals, Classified by Adult Bed Capacity, for 1956

Capacity in Adult Beds	No. of Hospitals	No. of Beds	Av. Daily Census*	Annual Admissions*
Under 25	925	15,724	8,425	558,167
25–49	1,635	57,490	33,889	1,849,642
50–99	1,611	109,391	73,435	3,410,903
100–199	1,249	173,497	128,558	5,299,196
200–299	571	137,098	106,054	4,002,117
300–499	433	162,911	127,837	3,816,611
500 and over	542	951,581	877,594	3,153,083
Total	6,966	1,607,692	1,355,792	22,089,719

* Estimated.

12

hospitals. Almost 80 per cent of the hospitals have less than 200 beds and more than one third have under 50 beds. This is true despite the fact that small hospitals usually cannot operate as efficiently as their larger counterparts and is the result of both local pride and the natural desire on the part of the public to have adequate hospital care close at hand.

As a contrast, nearly 60 per cent of the total hospital beds are contained in hospitals having 500 beds or more, even though institutions in this size-group make up less than 8 per cent of all hospitals. Over one half of the "500 beds or more" hospitals specialize in the care and treatment of psychiatric patients.

In 1956 the average capacity of all hospitals in the United States was 231 beds. General hospitals averaged 127 beds; psychiatric and tuberculosis hospitals, 1340 and 223 beds, respectively.

Average Length of Patient Stay. Another means of classifying hospitals is by average length of patient stay or, in other words, by their patients' average period of hospitalization. Under such a classification, hospitals are divided into "short-term" and "long-term" institutions. The average stay of patients in short-term hospitals is thirty days or less. Long-term hospitals, on the other hand, have an average patient stay exceeding thirty days.

Although completely accurate statistics are not available, it is estimated that more than four out of every five hospitals in this country are short-term institutions and that these hospitals account for approximately 97 per cent of all patient admissions.

Long-term hospitals, however, contain almost 57 per cent of the total hospital beds and about 62 per cent of all patients hospitalized in the United States on any given day. Almost all of the short-term institutions are general hospitals. Of the long-term hospitals, 43 per cent are psychiatric facilities, 26 per cent are tuberculosis institutions, and the remainder are general and "other special" hospitals.

Geographic Location. Still another method of classifying hospitals is by their geographic location. Governmental units, such as states and counties, often serve as the basis for a classification of this kind. More commonly, however, the various states and the hospitals they contain are grouped into regions. The regional classification adopted by the American Hospital Association and the states included in each region are listed below:

New England: Maine, New Hampshire, Vermont, Massachusetts, Rhode Island, Connecticut

Middle Atlantic: New York, New Jersey, Pennsylvania

South Atlantic: Delaware, Maryland, District of Columbia, Virginia, West Virginia, North Carolina, South Carolina, Georgia, Florida

East North Central: Ohio, Indiana, Illinois, Michigan, Wisconsin
East South Central: Kentucky, Tennessee, Alabama, Mississippi
West North Central: Minnesota, Iowa, Missouri, North Dakota, South
   Dakota, Nebraska, Kansas
West South Central: Arkansas, Louisiana, Oklahoma, Texas
Mountain: Montana, Idaho, Wyoming, Colorado, New Mexico, Ari-
   zona, Utah, Nevada
Pacific: Washington, Oregon, California

Table 4 depicts the variance among these regions in the number of hospitals and beds they contain and illustrates their relative importance to each other and to the total hospital industry.

Naturally, the number of hospitals and beds in each region is largely dependent on the regional population. As a result, the East North Central region, which has the greatest population, also has the most hospitals and is second in the number of hospital beds. The Middle Atlantic region has the largest number of beds and ranks second in population and hospitals. At the other extreme, the Mountain region has the smallest population and the fewest hospitals and beds.

Hospitals in the central and western regions are, on the average, much smaller than hospitals located in other areas of the country. One apparent reason for this variance is that the eastern part of the United States was settled first and hospitals in this section are therefore generally older and have had an opportunity to grow and develop. A second reason is that most of the central and western states cover vast land areas and yet, with several exceptions, have comparatively small, scattered populations. Large hospitals are impractical in such sparsely populated states, except in the metropolitan centers, because of the travel distances involved. Consequently, in some states many small institutions are necessary to provide the population with adequate hospital care and, in some instances, local feelings of independence tend to demand a unit of some size regardless of necessity.

There is a somewhat greater proportion of special hospitals and beds — other than psychiatric or tuberculosis — in the five regions east of the Mississippi than in the four western regions. This is particularly true of the New England, Middle Atlantic, and South Atlantic regions, which together contain more than one half of all maternity, orthopedic, contagious disease, chronic and convalescent, and eye, ear, nose and throat beds. Again, the eastern part of the country was settled first, and many of these hospitals were established at a time when specialized facilities were deemed more necessary than at present.

Among the individual states, the number of hospital beds generally correlates, as might be expected, with the population. New York, the most populous state, has by far the greatest number of hospital beds

Table 4. Comparative Analysis of Continental United States Hospitals, Classified by Geographic Region, for 1956

Geographic Region	No. of Hospitals	No. of Beds	Av. Daily Census*	Annual Admissions*	No. of Paid Personnel*†	Assets*	Annual Expenses*	Annual Payroll Expenses*
New England	439	122,177	101,614	1,340,150	111,261	$ 1,148,083,000	$ 488,275,000	$ 324,382,000
Middle Atlantic	1,003	400,731	354,827	4,106,375	322,244	3,462,686,000	1,397,392,000	921,638,000
South Atlantic	905	201,706	167,879	3,165,723	178,124	1,681,661,000	734,301,000	467,998,000
East North Central ...	1,215	326,519	284,357	4,503,658	270,380	2,557,471,000	1,238,549,000	812,771,000
East South Central ...	525	87,817	70,502	1,460,115	71,961	589,853,000	284,147,000	179,503,000
West North Central ...	887	138,556	110,444	2,093,101	119,815	1,045,847,000	502,520,000	328,157,000
West South Central ...	908	118,792	93,249	2,203,051	104,902	885,627,000	487,985,000	275,361,000
Mountain	431	53,288	41,469	927,650	52,359	456,393,000	225,453,000	149,496,000
Pacific	653	158,106	131,451	2,289,896	143,658	1,207,947,000	708,237,000	489,631,000
Total	6,966	1,607,692	1,355,792	22,089,719	1,374,704	$13,035,068,000	$6,016,859,000	$3,948,937,000

* Estimated.
† Includes full-time personnel plus full-time equivalents of part-time personnel.

Patterns of Hospital Ownership and Control

Table 5. Comparison of Governmental and Nongovernmental Hospitals with All
Continental United States Hospitals in 1956

	All Continental U.S. Hospitals	% of U.S. Total	Gov. Hospitals	% of U.S. Total	Nongov. Hospitals	% of U.S. Total
Number of hospitals	6,966	100.0	2,248	32.3	4,718	67.7
Number of beds..	1,607,692	100.0	1,114,640	69.3	493,050	30.7
Average daily census	1,355,792	100.0	992,265	73.1	363,527	26.9
Annual admissions	22,089,719	100.0	5,718,632	25.9	16,371,087	74.1
Number of paid personnel	1,374,704	100.0	648,835	47.2	725,869	52.8
Assets	$13,035,068,000	100.0	$6,570,464,000	50.4	$6,464,614,000	49.6
Annual expenses..	$ 6,016,859,000	100.0	$2,894,106,000	48.1	$3,122,753,000	51.9
Annual payroll expenses	$ 3,948,937,000	100.0	$2,060,277,000	52.2	$1,888,660,000	47.8

and is followed by California, Pennsylvania, Illinois, and Ohio, which also rank second, third, fourth, and fifth, respectively, in population. The number of hospitals contained in the various states is also related to population; however, the correlation is not as exact as with hospital beds. Texas, for example, has the most hospitals, with 561 such institutions, and yet ranks sixth in population and eighth in number of hospital beds.

At the other extreme, Nevada has both the smallest population and the fewest hospital beds. Delaware, which ranks forty-fifth in population, has seventeen hospitals, less than any other state.

Ownership and Control. By far the greater number of hospitals in this country are both operated and controlled by their legal owners. However, in some hospitals ownership is vested in one organization and control of operation in another. An example of the latter is the national leprosarium at Carville, Louisiana, which is owned by the United States Public Health Service, an agency of the federal government, but which is operated by a religious order of the Roman Catholic Church.

Hospitals, according to the ownership and control classification, may be divided into governmental and nongovernmental institutions. Table 5 illustrates the importance of these two divisions in relation to each other and to the total hospital industry.

The above categories may, in turn, be subdivided into smaller groups and finally into individual patterns. The description of these smaller groups and of the individual patterns is the major purpose of this study and is the basis of all the subsequent chapters.

PART I · GOVERNMENTAL PATTERNS

Healing is a matter of time, but it is sometimes also a matter of opportunity.   HIPPOCRATES

The health of the people is really the foundation upon which all their happiness and all their powers as a State depend.   BENJAMIN DISRAELI

Governmental Hospitals and Their Significance

GOVERNMENTAL hospitals are owned and operated by agencies or departments of the federal, state, and local governments. They constitute less than one third of the nation's total hospitals and admit just over one fourth of all hospital patients; however, they contain more than two thirds of the hospital beds in this country. In addition, these governmental facilities account for approximately one half of all hospital assets, expenses, and personnel. (See Table 6.)

This chapter briefly summarizes the total significance of federal, state, and local governmental hospitals. A more detailed discussion of hospitals operated by individual federal agencies, state governments, and different units of local government follows in subsequent chapters.

FEDERAL HOSPITALS

The citizens of the United States are becoming increasingly dependent on the central government for certain basic services. This is particularly evident in the field of public health. As an example, over thirty million people are either currently eligible or may, in the future, become eligible to receive hospital, medical, and dental care at federal expense. Among the real and potential beneficiaries of such care are (1) veterans of military service; (2) armed forces personnel and retired personnel; (3) dependents of military personnel; (4) civilian employees of the federal government for accidents or illnesses incurred in the "line of duty"; (5) American Indians and Eskimos; (6) American merchant seamen; (7) Coast Guard personnel and their dependents; (8) inmates of federal penitentiaries; (9) the civilian population of the Panama Canal Zone; (10) narcotic addicts; (11) lepers.

In addition to providing services to the above groups, the central government beneficially influences the nation's health in other ways. Federal funds aid the various states in obtaining the necessities of life,

19

Table 6. Comparison of Governmental Hospitals with All
Continental United States Hospitals in 1956

	Gov. Total	% of U.S. Total
Number of hospitals	2,248	32.3
Number of beds	1,114,640	69.3
Average daily census	992,265	73.1
Annual admissions	5,718,632	25.9
Number of paid personnel	648,835	47.2
Assets	$6,570,464,000	50.4
Annual expenses	$2,894,106,000	48.1
Annual payroll expenses	$2,060,277,000	52.2

including health services, for public assistance cases such as dependent children, the aged, the blind, and the permanently and totally disabled. Also, under the terms of the Hospital Survey and Construction Act (Hill-Burton), federal funds are available, on a matching basis, for the construction of nonfederal hospital facilities.

Three different methods are employed by the federal government in providing hospital, medical, and dental care to eligible beneficiaries in the groups enumerated above: (1) contracting with private organizations to operate federally-owned hospitals; (2) direct purchase of hospital, medical, and dental care from private hospitals, clinics, physicians, and dentists; (3) furnishing the services in federally owned and operated hospitals, clinics and dispensaries.

The first method is normally used where the provision of hospital care is an adjunct community facility essential to the accomplishment of some major and fundamental program of a federal agency. For example, the Atomic Energy Commission contracts with private corporations to operate and maintain all government-owned community facilities, including hospitals, at its research centers in Tennessee, New Mexico, and Washington. Other federal agencies, such as the National Park Service, provide health services under similar contractual relationships.

In 1956 the federal government expended approximately $110 million in direct purchase of hospital, medical, and dental care from private sources. Of this amount, over 60 per cent was for services rendered to dependents of military personnel under the "Medicare" program. Another sizable portion, nearly 30 per cent, was expended for the care of veterans. Even though it operates its own facilities, the Veterans Administration is making extensive use of nonfederal hospitals and private medical and dental consultants in serving its beneficiaries.

The federally owned and operated facilities, referred to above in the central government's third method of providing health services, constitute what is often called "the federal hospital system." The significance of federal hospitals in comparison with all governmental hospitals and the total hospital industry is shown in Table 7.

Approximately 94 per cent of the continental federal hospitals and beds are operated by five agencies — the Veterans Administration, the three armed services of the Department of Defense, and the United States Public Health Service of the Department of Health, Education, and Welfare — each of which is discussed individually in subsequent chapters.

Table 7. Comparison of Federal Hospitals with Governmental Hospitals and
All Continental United States Hospitals in 1956

	Federal Total	% of Gov. Total	% of U.S. Total
Number of hospitals	432	19.2	6.2
Number of beds	184,121	16.5	11.4
Average daily census*	156,192	15.7	11.5
Annual admissions*	1,388,307	24.3	6.3
Number of paid personnel*	197,892	30.5	14.4
Assets*	$1,902,528,000	29.0	14.6
Annual expenses*	$ 967,651,000	33.4	16.1
Annual payroll expenses*	$ 783,341,000	38.0	19.9

Note: Data pertains only to those federal hospitals in the continental United States. Infirmaries, dispensaries, and overseas hospitals are excluded from this table.
* Estimated.

Included in the remaining 6 per cent are (1) the hospital units of federal penitentiaries and correctional institutions, operated by the Bureau of Prisons of the Department of Justice and professionally staffed by the United States Public Health Service; (2) Freedmen's Hospital in Washington, D.C., an institution staffed entirely by Negroes, which is semi-autonomous but organizationally is under the United States Public Health Service; and (3) St. Elizabeth's Hospital, also in the nation's capital, a large neuropsychiatric institution under the direct control of the Department of Health, Education, and Welfare.

The Bureau of the Budget, a division of the Executive Office of the President of the United States, reviews and coordinates all federal hospital, convalescent, and domiciliary programs to (1) avoid duplication of services and overbuilding of facilities; (2) ensure the most efficient and complete utilization of the total services and facilities of the federal government; (3) appraise the need for existing or additional facilities; (4) bring about the maximum utilization of nonfederal facilities in the administration of the hospital activities or programs of federal agencies.

STATE GOVERNMENTAL HOSPITALS

Hospitals owned and maintained by state governments represent one of the most important patterns of hospital ownership and control. With the general exception of state university hospitals and hospital departments of state schools and correctional institutions, the control of state governmental hospitals normally rests with departments, boards, or administrative agencies of the state governments.

As illustrated in Table 8, in 1956 nearly 8 per cent of all hospitals in the United States and approximately 25 per cent of the governmental hospitals were state institutions. Even more significant is the fact that in that year state hospitals contained more than 45 per cent of all hospital beds in this country and over 65 per cent of all governmental hospital beds.

In 1956 the total of 553 state governmental hospitals included 271 state psychiatric institutions. The most important phase of state governmental hospital care is in the field of mental illness. This is best indicated by the fact that in that year state psychiatric institutions contained over 90 per cent of the beds in all state hospitals and more than 86 per cent of the beds in all psychiatric hospitals in the United States. In addition to providing almost all of the institutional care to the mentally ill in the United States, a high proportion of hospital care was furnished by state governmental hospitals to tuberculosis patients.

The significance of all state governmental hospitals in comparison with all governmental hospitals and the total hospital industry is shown in Table 8.

Table 8. Comparison of State Governmental Hospitals with Governmental Hospitals and All Continental United States Hospitals in 1956

	State Gov. Total	% of Gov. Total	% of U.S. Total
Number of hospitals	553	24.6	7.9
Number of beds........................	728,151	65.3	45.3
Average daily census *	681,000	68.6	50.2
Annual admissions *	861,000	15.1	3.9
Number of paid personnel *	243,180	37.5	17.7
Assets *	$2,500,000,000	38.5	19.2
Annual expenses *	$1,044,000,000	36.1	17.3
Annual payroll expenses *	$ 668,000,000	3.2	1.7

* Estimated.

LOCAL GOVERNMENTAL HOSPITALS

Local governmental hospitals are owned and operated by individual units of local government or by a combination of two or more such units. They include district, county, city-county, and city hospitals, each of which will be discussed individually in the chapter on state and local governmental hospitals. Together, these institutions represent an extremely important source of hospital care in the United States (see Table 9). This is illustrated by the fact that they account for 18 per cent of all hospitals, 13 per cent of all hospital beds, and 16 per cent of all hospital admissions. In addition, they constitute 56 per cent of all governmental hospitals, contain 18 per cent of all governmental hospital beds, and provide care to 61 per cent of all patients admitted to governmental hospitals.

Table 9. Comparison of Local Governmental Hospitals with Governmental Hospitals and All Continental United States Hospitals in 1956

	Loc. Gov. Total	% of Gov. Total	% of U.S. Total
Number of hospitals	1,263	56.2	18.1
Number of beds	202,368	18.2	12.6
Average daily census *	157,000	15.8	11.6
Annual admissions *	3,500,000	61.2	15.8
Number of paid personnel *	231,000	35.6	16.8
Assets *	$1,800,000,000	27.4	13.8
Annual expenses *	$ 986,000,000	34.1	16.4
Annual payroll expenses *	$ 665,000,000	32.3	16.8

* Estimated.

However, local governmental hospitals have a much greater effect on the hospital industry in this country than that represented by the above statistics. They provide a high proportion of the total hospital care rendered to the medically indigent in the United States and, in addition, they include some of the finest hospitals in the world for the education and clinical training of medical students, interns, and residents. Also, most of the "emergency" hospitals in metropolitan centers are local governmental institutions.

Many of these institutions are plagued by political interference and inadequate financial support. In addition, our booming economy since the end of World War II and the phenomenal growth of the various health insurance plans in recent years have considerably reduced the indigent and medically indigent population. Another factor contributing to the lessening need for local governmental hospitals is the emerging policy of local governments to disperse indigent patients among local voluntary hospitals and to pay for their care. As a result, many of the local governmental hospitals which were established principally to serve the medically indigent are presently lacking patients and are finding it difficult to justify their continued existence.

Although seemingly contradictory, the local governmental hospital pattern has shown an over-all increase in the past ten to twenty years in both hospitals and beds. Furthermore, despite the many problems, influences, and lessening need, it appears that the number of city, county, and city-county hospitals and beds will remain at a fairly constant level in the future because of political pressures to maintain a party machine through job opportunities coupled with union pressures to wield strong influence on wage levels and job continuance. Another important factor is the eagerness of medical schools to maintain their sources of teaching patients. As a result, these various pressures and influences will cause most of the local governmental institutions to be continued by changing the scope of local hospital services and the types of patients served.

Federal Hospitals

Two types of hospitals, fixed and nonfixed, are maintained by the Department of the Army. Fixed hospitals are designed to operate in the same location over an extended period of time. Nonfixed hospitals are mobile and designed to provide close medical support for combat elements. However, regardless of their location, mission, size, type, or bed capacity, all Army hospitals are similar in their organization and administration.

Hospitals located outside the continental limits of the United States, its territories or possessions, are under the jurisdiction of the overseas theater commanders. They are generally designated both by number and as surgical, evacuation, field, station, general, or convalescent hospital centers.

Army hospitals in the United States are usually of the fixed type and designated as either Class I or Class II hospitals. The remainder of this chapter will, for the most part, be limited to a discussion of these two classes of Army hospitals.

Class I hospitals are the most numerous and are generally established at the forts, camps, depots, and other military facilities operated by the Army. Normally, they are under the jurisdiction of the commanders of the Army areas in which they are located.

Class II hospitals are under the command jurisdiction of the Surgeon General of the Army. They include such well-known Army hospitals and medical centers as Walter Reed, Brooke, Fitzsimons, Letterman, and Valley Forge.

Organizational Structure and Governing Authority. The Department of the Army functions as part of the Department of Defense (see Figs. 1 and 2). The Secretary of the Army, subject to the general direction and control of the President of the United States and the Secretary of Defense, is responsible for the conduct of all Army affairs and exercises immediate control over the Department of the Army.

Figure 1. Office of the Secretary of Defense, 1956

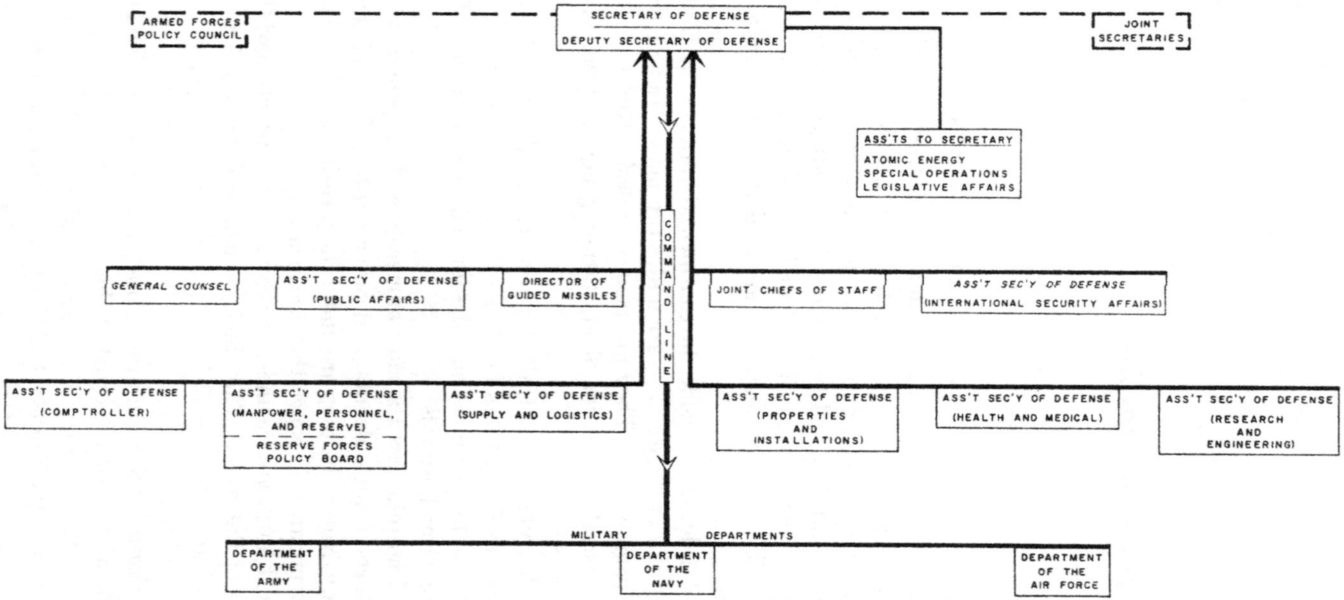

ARMED FORCES POLICY COUNCIL

JOINT SECRETARIES

SECRETARY OF DEFENSE
DEPUTY SECRETARY OF DEFENSE

ASS'TS TO SECRETARY
ATOMIC ENERGY
SPECIAL OPERATIONS
LEGISLATIVE AFFAIRS

JOINT CHIEFS OF STAFF

ASS'T SEC'Y OF DEFENSE (INTERNATIONAL SECURITY AFFAIRS)

ASS'T SEC'Y OF DEFENSE (RESEARCH AND ENGINEERING)

ASS'T SEC'Y OF DEFENSE (PROPERTIES AND INSTALLATIONS)

ASS'T SEC'Y OF DEFENSE (HEALTH AND MEDICAL)

DIRECTOR OF GUIDED MISSILES

ASS'T SEC'Y OF DEFENSE (SUPPLY AND LOGISTICS)

ASS'T SEC'Y OF DEFENSE (PUBLIC AFFAIRS)

GENERAL COUNSEL

ASS'T SEC'Y OF DEFENSE (MANPOWER, PERSONNEL, AND RESERVE)
RESERVE FORCES POLICY BOARD

ASS'T SEC'Y OF DEFENSE (COMPTROLLER)

COMMAND LINE

MILITARY DEPARTMENTS

DEPARTMENT OF THE ARMY

DEPARTMENT OF THE NAVY

DEPARTMENT OF THE AIR FORCE

26

Figure 2. Department of the Army, 1956

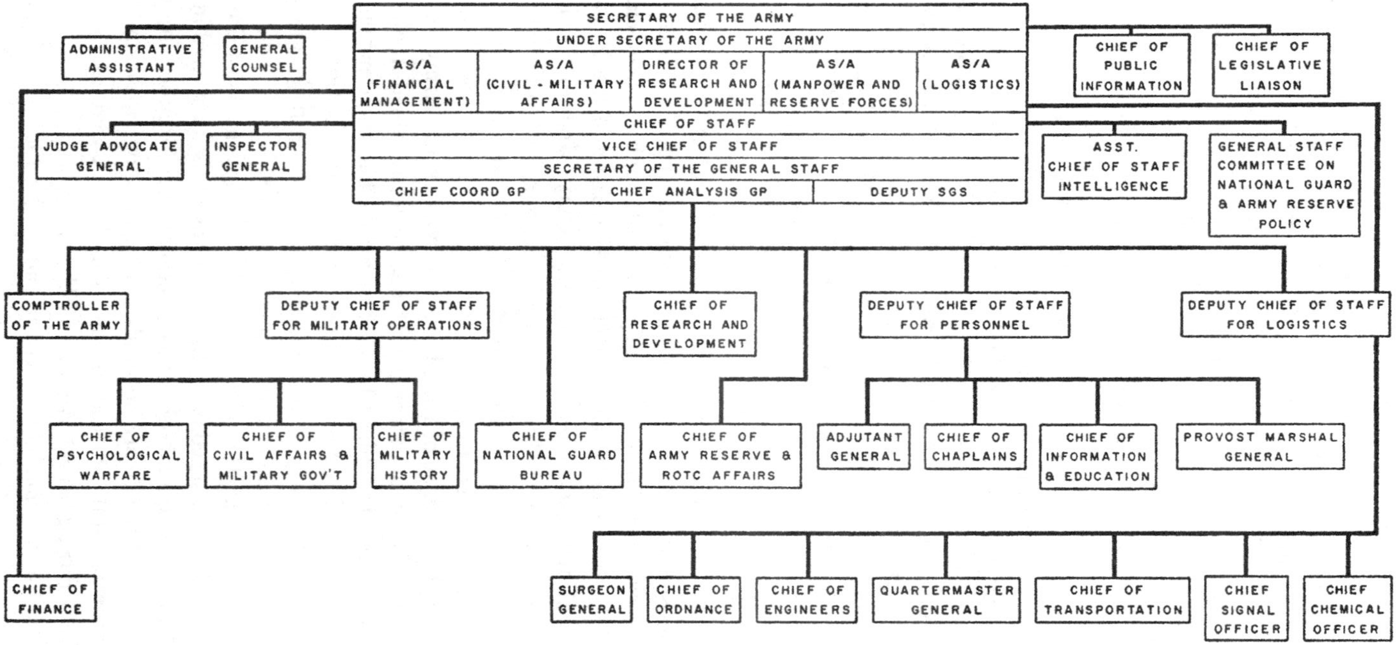

27

Patterns of Hospital Ownership and Control

The Chief of Staff is the principal military advisor to the Secretary of the Army. He is directly responsible to the Secretary for the efficiency of the Army and its state of preparedness for military operations.

The Deputy Chief of Staff for Logistics, under the functional supervision of the Assistant Secretary of the Army (Logistics) and under the direct supervision and control of the Chief of Staff, is responsible for the activities of the technical services, including the Army Medical Service.

The Surgeon General of the Army is appointed for a four-year period and holds the rank of Major General. He supervises the Army Medical Service and assists and advises the Chief of Staff and the Secretary of the Army on health and medical matters (see Fig. 3).

Admission Requirements. The hospitalization of all Army personnel and of all other persons authorized to receive care under certain circumstances and conditions is governed by statutory authority and Army regulations. Hospital commanders have jurisdiction over the admission of patients to their institutions. Medical and hospital care may be provided eligible patients who are *not* members of a uniformed service if space, facilities, and staff are available. However, the primary mission of the various Army medical facilities is to render service to Army personnel and members of the other uniformed services. The care provided nonmilitary patients must not interfere with this mission and must not exceed the care furnished uniformed services personnel.

History of Growth and Development. Although it was officially established as the Hospital Department of the Army of the Revolution by the Continental Congress in 1775, the Army Medical Service at first existed only in time of war or threatened war. Not until 1818 did Congress authorize a Surgeon General and a Medical Service as a permanent part of the Army.

The rightful place of the Medical Service in the Army environment has been difficult to determine. It has been revamped in almost every war or conflict in which the United States has been engaged and, in addition, has undergone several peacetime reorganizations. The responsibilities of the Surgeon General and his position in the chain of command have also changed at frequent intervals.

The hospital at the U.S. Military Academy at West Point is the oldest of the present continental Army hospitals. It opened in 1826 and was followed a year later by the hospital at Fort Monroe, Virginia. However, most of the Army hospitals currently in operation in the United States were established after the turn of the twentieth century, particularly during World Wars I and II.

Measures of Significance. At the end of the 1958 fiscal year, the De-

Figure 3. Office of the Surgeon General, 1956

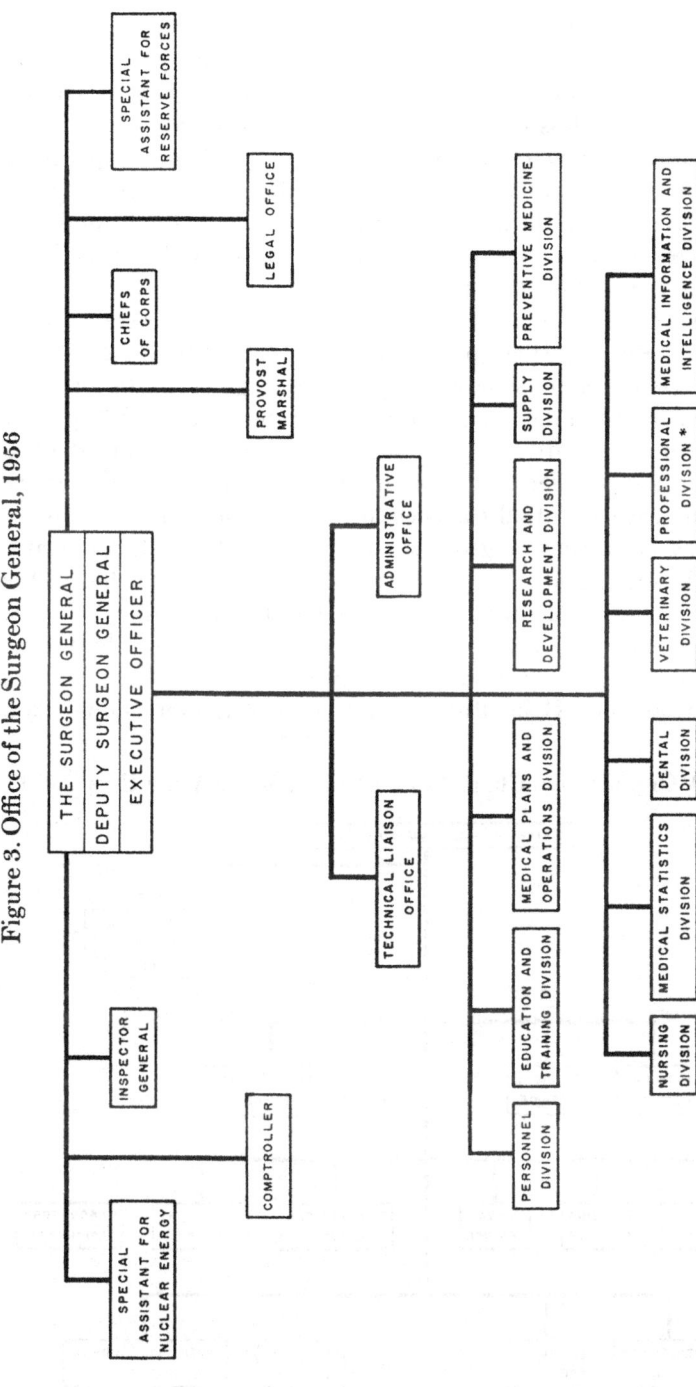

* Includes nine chief consultants: medicine; pathology and allied sciences; physical medicine; psychiatry and neurology; radiology; surgery; physical standards; special services; pharmacy.

29

partment of the Army was maintaining fifty-seven hospitals within the continental limits of the United States with a capacity of 14,590 operating beds. Eight of these institutions were Class II hospitals and the remainder were Class I installations (see Figs. 4 and 5).

Overseas, there were approximately thirty-one Army hospitals with a capacity of around 6800 operating beds. However, completely accurate information on the hospital installations outside the United States was not readily available and the following statistical data pertains primarily to the *continental* Army hospitals.

During the 1958 fiscal year, about 300,000 patients were estimated to have been admitted to the fifty-seven continental hospitals, or roughly twenty admissions per bed. An average of 10,200 beds were occupied daily and the average occupancy rate was around 70 per cent.

Army hospitals are generally larger than those maintained by the Air Force and smaller than those operated by the Navy. The average operating capacity of all continental Army hospitals in 1958 approximated 255 beds. They ranged in size from the five-bed installation at the Black Hills Ordnance Depot in Provo, South Dakota, to the 1250-bed Walter Reed Army Hospital in Washington, D. C. Typically, the Class II hospitals have a greater capacity than the Class I installations. Almost one half of the continental Army hospital beds were contained in the eight Class II institutions. Only four of the forty-nine Class I

Figure 4. Organization Chart, Class I United States Army Hospital, 1956

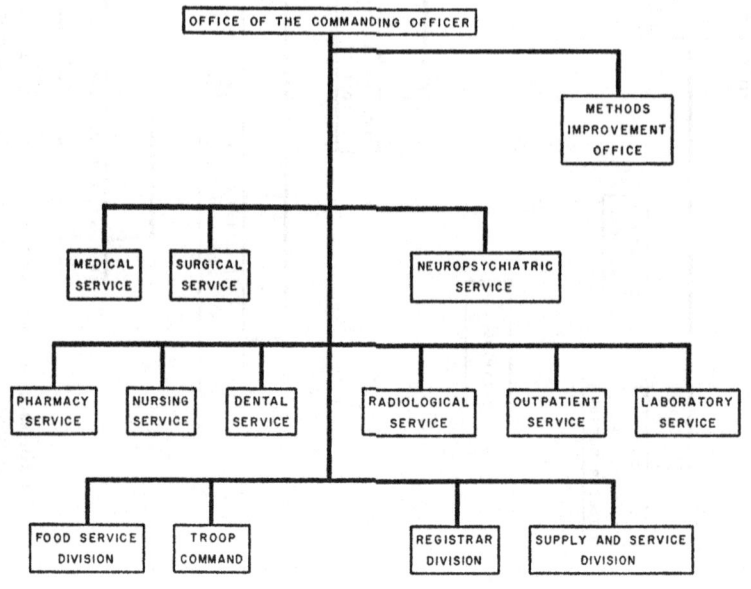

Figure 5. Organization Chart, Class II United States Army Hospital, 1956

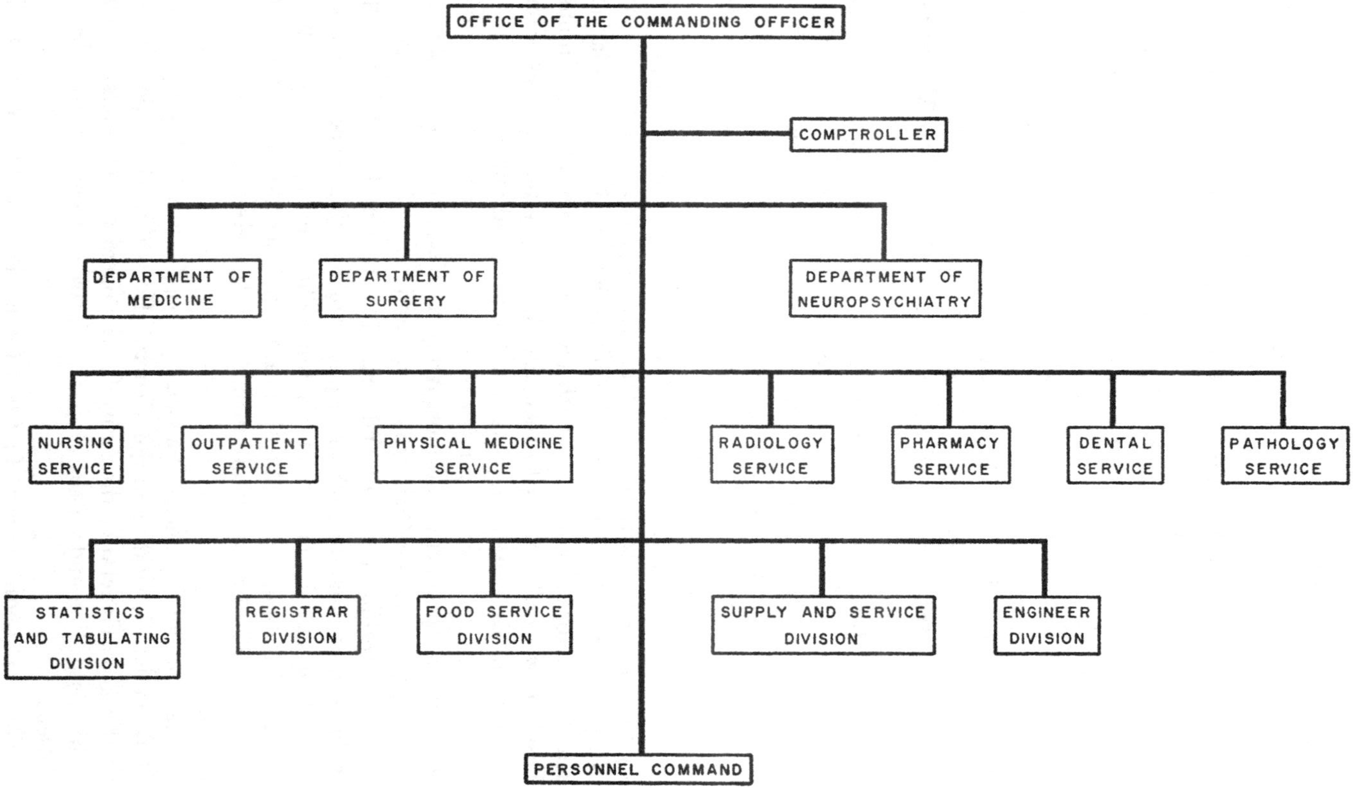

OFFICE OF THE COMMANDING OFFICER

COMPTROLLER

DEPARTMENT OF MEDICINE

DEPARTMENT OF SURGERY

DEPARTMENT OF NEUROPSYCHIATRY

NURSING SERVICE

OUTPATIENT SERVICE

PHYSICAL MEDICINE SERVICE

RADIOLOGY SERVICE

PHARMACY SERVICE

DENTAL SERVICE

PATHOLOGY SERVICE

STATISTICS AND TABULATING DIVISION

REGISTRAR DIVISION

FOOD SERVICE DIVISION

SUPPLY AND SERVICE DIVISION

ENGINEER DIVISION

PERSONNEL COMMAND

hospitals had more than 500 operating beds while two of the eight Class II installations contained 1000 or more beds.

As of July 1958, forty-seven Army hospitals — forty-one in the United States and six overseas — had been accredited by the Joint Commission on Accreditation of Hospitals. The Department of the Army also reported in July 1958 that twenty-one continental and two overseas hospitals were members of the American Hospital Association. Only six continental Army hospitals belonged to state and/or regional hospital associations.

Army hospitals are well dispersed throughout the United States; each of the nine geographic regions contained at least one such institution in 1958. Most of the Class II hospitals were located in the western part of the country, particularly the Southwest, while the Class I installations were distributed in equal numbers east and west of the Mississippi River.

Financial Data. Although accurate figures were not available, continental Army hospitals were estimated to have expended in excess of $100 million in the 1958 fiscal year. Total assets of the same institutions were estimated at more than $200 million.

Congressional appropriations are the principal source of both operating income and capital funds.

Educational Activities. Twelve Army hospitals had been approved by the American Medical Association for residency training in 1958. Nine hospitals were approved for internships and two installations maintained formal affiliations with medical schools. Three additional hospitals were affiliated with such schools on an informal basis. None of the hospitals operated a professional or practical nursing school.

The Army conducts a number of specialist courses in the various paramedical specialties, and most Army hospitals maintain on-the-job training programs for their professional and nonprofessional personnel.

Administration. The command element of an Army hospital generally includes a commanding officer, deputy commanding officer (when assigned), executive officer, and adjutant. The commander and deputy commander are officers in the Medical Corps (medical), while the executive officer and adjutant are members of the Medical Service Corps (nonmedical).

The commanding officer of a Class II hospital usually holds the rank of Brigadier General or Major General. He is directly responsible to the Surgeon General of the Army for the operation and management of his institution and for the professional care and services provided to patients.

The commanding officer of a Class I Army hospital also serves in the capacity of post surgeon. Normally, he holds the rank of Colonel and is directly responsible for hospital operation to the commander of the post on which the hospital is located.

The deputy commanding officer in either a Class I or Class II installation understudies the commanding officer and serves as his principal assistant, particularly in the area of professional services. When a deputy commanding officer is not assigned, the commanding officer may appoint a senior Medical Corps officer to serve, in addition to his other duties, as Chief of Professional Services to assist in coordinating professional matters.

The executive officer in either a Class I or Class II hospital is the principal assistant and advisor to the commanding officer on administrative matters. The adjutant assists the executive officer in carrying out his administrative duties.

Medical Staff. The medical staff of an Army hospital is organized by clinical services. Professional activities are coordinated by the deputy commanding officer, or in the absence of a deputy commander, by the senior Medical Corps officer appointed by the hospital commander to serve as Chief of Professional Services.

As of May 1958, there were over 4000 physicians in the Army Medical Corps.

Trends. Although a number of Army hospitals have been established since the end of World War II, the medical facilities of the Army are apparently near their peacetime peak. The current construction program is primarily designed to replace and renovate old, obsolete institutions rather than to increase the number of hospitals and beds. The future size of the hospital system operated by the Department of the Army is naturally contingent on the number of personnel that will be required to fulfill the ever-changing role and mission of the Army. However, unless war breaks out, the number of Army hospitals and beds should remain relatively constant in the coming years.

UNITED STATES NAVAL HOSPITALS

The Bureau of Medicine and Surgery of the Department of the Navy is responsible for safeguarding the health of the Navy and Marine Corps and is charged with the operation and maintenance of all United States naval hospitals.

The term "naval hospital" is applied to those hospital installations of the Navy which are self-contained command units under the direct operating control of the Surgeon General of the Navy as the Chief, Bureau of Medicine and Surgery. The following discussion pertains primarily to "naval" hospitals and only occasionally applies to the various station hospitals and dispensaries which are also maintained by the Navy but which are not self-contained command units.

Patterns of Hospital Ownership and Control

The primary mission of a naval hospital includes (1) the care and treatment of sick and injured military personnel with the object of their expeditious return to duty; (2) the prompt disposition of patients who require very prolonged forms of treatment or who are found physically unfit for retention in the military service; (3) the care and treatment of dependents of active duty and retired military personnel.

The secondary mission of a naval hospital includes the instruction of all Medical Department personnel, including intern and resident training; the care and treatment of other authorized nonmilitary patients; research in medicine, dentistry, and related specialties; and cooperation with military and civilian authorities in matters pertaining to health, sanitation, local disasters, emergencies, and catastrophies.

Organizational Structure and Governing Authority. The Department of the Navy is subject to the general direction and control of the President of the United States and the Secretary of Defense. Immediate direction and control is exercised by the Secretary of the Navy, who has general supervision of all naval affairs (see Fig. 6). The various naval bureaus — including the Bureau of Medicine and Surgery — are directed by the Under Secretary of the Navy.

The Chief, Bureau of Medicine and Surgery (Fig. 7), is designated as the Surgeon General of the Navy. Appointed for a four-year period, he holds the rank of Rear Admiral. The Surgeon General is responsible to the Under Secretary of the Navy and thus to the Secretary of the Navy for the operation of the Bureau, including the operation and management of all naval hospitals. In addition, he serves as a technical advisor in that field to the Secretary of the Navy.

Admission Requirements. Naval regulations and statutory authority cover the hospitalization and treatment of all categories of naval personnel and of all other persons authorized, under certain circumstances, to receive care. Admission to naval hospitals depends upon the category of personnel applying for or requiring admission and the availability of facilities and personnel to provide the necessary care. Some nonmilitary personnel categories cannot be admitted for certain specified chronic conditions and must seek hospitalization and treatment from other sources. In general, admission to a naval hospital is made on the recommendation of a naval medical officer. Humanitarian cases may be admitted at the discretion of the commanding officer of an individual hospital.

Dependents of active duty or retired military personnel are billed $1.75 per day for subsistence while receiving inpatient medical care in Army, Navy, or Air Force hospitals. Under the terms of the Dependents' Medical Care Act, dependents of active duty personnel may elect to enter civilian hospitals where they are charged $1.75 per day or

Figure 6. Department of the Navy, 1956

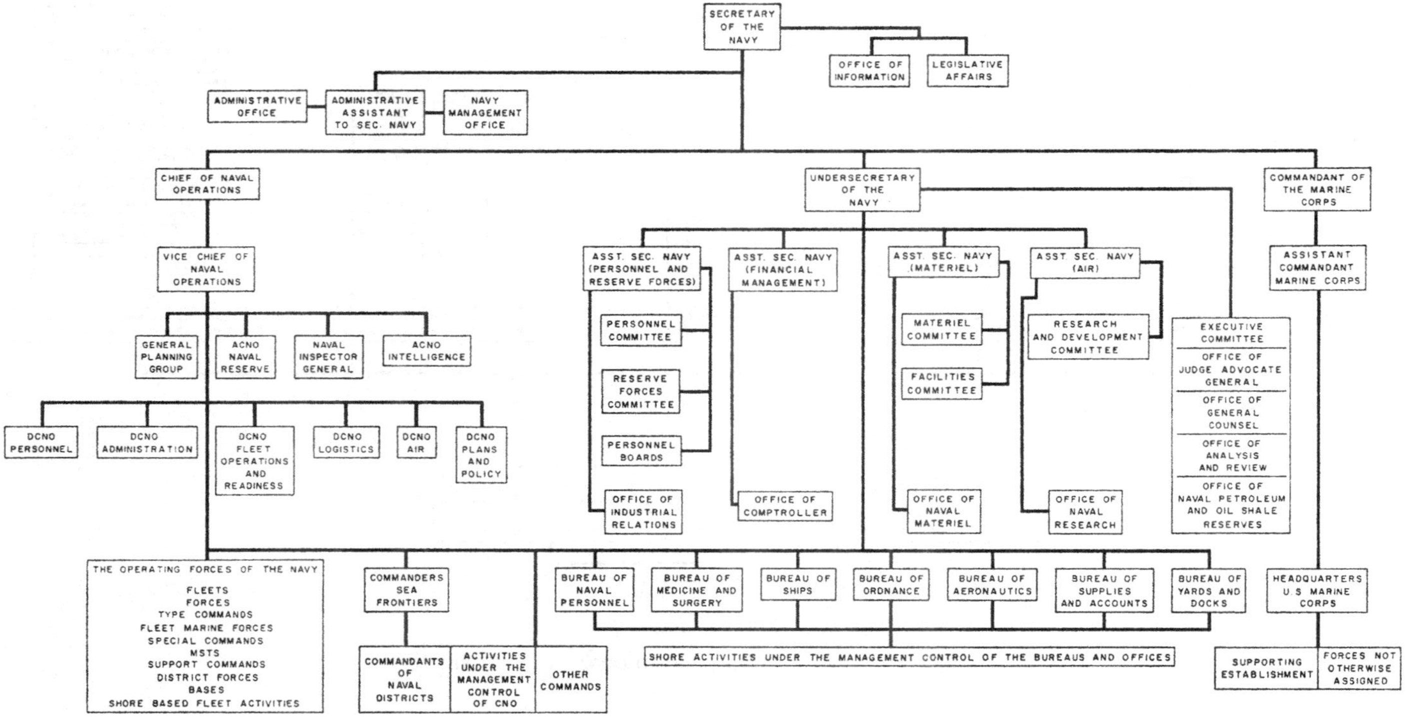

Figure 7. Bureau of Medicine and Surgery, 1956

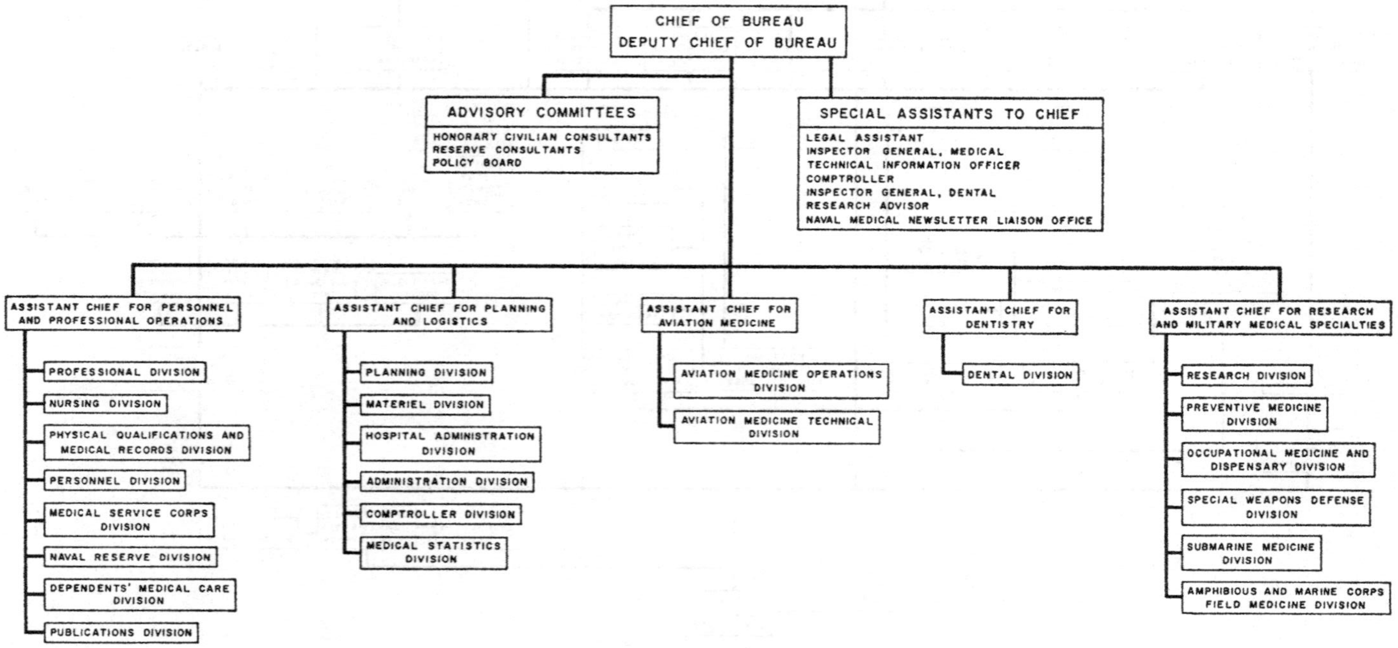

CHIEF OF BUREAU
DEPUTY CHIEF OF BUREAU

SPECIAL ASSISTANTS TO CHIEF
LEGAL ASSISTANT
INSPECTOR GENERAL, MEDICAL
TECHNICAL INFORMATION OFFICER
COMPTROLLER
INSPECTOR GENERAL, DENTAL
RESEARCH ADVISOR
NAVAL MEDICAL NEWSLETTER LIAISON OFFICE

ADVISORY COMMITTEES
HONORARY CIVILIAN CONSULTANTS
RESERVE CONSULTANTS
POLICY BOARD

ASSISTANT CHIEF FOR PERSONNEL AND PROFESSIONAL OPERATIONS
- PROFESSIONAL DIVISION
- NURSING DIVISION
- PHYSICAL QUALIFICATIONS AND MEDICAL RECORDS DIVISION
- PERSONNEL DIVISION
- MEDICAL SERVICE CORPS DIVISION
- NAVAL RESERVE DIVISION
- DEPENDENTS' MEDICAL CARE DIVISION
- PUBLICATIONS DIVISION

ASSISTANT CHIEF FOR PLANNING AND LOGISTICS
- PLANNING DIVISION
- MATERIEL DIVISION
- HOSPITAL ADMINISTRATION DIVISION
- ADMINISTRATION DIVISION
- COMPTROLLER DIVISION
- MEDICAL STATISTICS DIVISION

ASSISTANT CHIEF FOR AVIATION MEDICINE
- AVIATION MEDICINE OPERATIONS DIVISION
- AVIATION MEDICINE TECHNICAL DIVISION

ASSISTANT CHIEF FOR DENTISTRY
- DENTAL DIVISION

ASSISTANT CHIEF FOR RESEARCH AND MILITARY MEDICAL SPECIALTIES
- RESEARCH DIVISION
- PREVENTIVE MEDICINE DIVISION
- OCCUPATIONAL MEDICINE AND DISPENSARY DIVISION
- SPECIAL WEAPONS DEFENSE DIVISION
- SUBMARINE MEDICINE DIVISION
- AMPHIBIOUS AND MARINE CORPS FIELD MEDICINE DIVISION

36

a total of $25.00, whichever is higher for a given period of hospitalization.

History of Growth and Development. Prior to the Revolutionary War, all seafaring men of the American colonies were required to pay a portion of their earnings to support the Greenwich Hospital in England for sick and disabled seamen. This support was, of course, discontinued in 1776 with the beginning of the war and the severing of relations between the United States and England.

Several attempts were made in the years immediately following the war's end to draft legislation providing for the hospitalization and medical relief of American merchant seamen. Not until 1798, however, was such a bill passed by Congress and signed by President John Adams. This bill, which created our present Public Health Service, provided for the construction of marine hospitals in coastal cities and authorized the deduction of twenty cents per month from the wages of each merchant seaman to finance the construction and to support the medical care program. In 1799 the bill was amended to include the officers and enlisted personnel of the Navy and Marine Corps.

During the following decade, naval personnel became extremely dissatisfied with the marine hospital system. In many ports, hospitals did not exist and the accommodations in the few hospitals that were maintained left much to be desired. Practically no naval officers and only a few of the enlisted personnel took advantage of the scanty provisions offered, and of those who did, three out of five deserted as soon as they had attained a sufficient degree of convalescence. At New York, the sick were housed in a rude structure in the Navy Yard which was described in 1810 as follows: "To give you some faint idea of what is called a hospital on this station, imagine to yourself an old mill situated on the margin of a millpond, where every high tide flows from 12 to 15 inches upon the low floor and there deposits a quantity of mud and sediment, and which has no other covering to protect the sick from the inclemency of the season than a common clapboard outside, without lining or ceiling on the inside. If, sir, you can figure to yourself such a place, you will have some idea of the situation of the sick on this station."

In 1811, Congress passed a law establishing a separate Naval Hospital Fund to be supported by the twenty cents per month deduction from the wages of all personnel together with all fines imposed on officers, seamen, and marines. The fund was augmented by $50,000 out of the unexpended balance of the Marine Hospital Fund and, in later years, additional revenue was received from forfeitures of pay because of desertion and from donations.

In 1827 the first permanent hospital installations were started at

37

Norfolk, Virginia, and Philadelphia, Pennsylvania. The Norfolk hospital opened in 1830, even though the building had not been completed, and the Philadelphia institution followed three years later. Four other naval hospitals were also established in the 1830s.

Naval hospitals increased tremendously in both size and number in World Wars I and II. During the latter conflict, the capacity of continental naval hospitals went from 8437 to 64,000 beds and a total of eighty-five hospitals were in commission. Many of these were established in hotels which had been taken over by the Navy. At one time during this period the hospital in San Diego had a census of more than 10,000 patients.

By 1950 the number of hospitals had been reduced to twenty-six. However, with the outbreak of hostilities in Korea, one additional hospital was commissioned and another was reactivated.

Measures of Significance. At the end of the 1958 fiscal year the United States Navy was again maintaining twenty-six naval hospitals — all of which were general-acute institutions — with a combined operating capacity of 15,725 beds. Twenty-three of the hospitals were located within the continental limits of the United States and three were overseas. The Navy was also maintaining thirty-one station hospitals, one hospital ship, and seventy-eight dispensaries.

During 1957, naval hospitals admitted 217,873 patients. The average daily census approximated 13,000 patients and the average occupancy rate exceeded 80 per cent.

In the same period, naval hospitals were staffed by more than 11,000 military and 7000 civilian personnel. Some of the personnel in naval hospitals perform functions for which there is no counterpart in nonmilitary hospitals, such as handling service records for both patients and staff and providing fire and police protection. As is true of all service hospitals, patient labor is utilized to a limited degree.

Unusually large naval hospitals had an average operating capacity of over 600 beds at the end of the 1958 fiscal year. The twenty-three hospitals in the United States ranged in size from a 50-bed installation in Bainbridge, Maryland to 2125 beds in the hospital at San Diego. Five of the continental hospitals had more than 1000 beds.

All continental naval hospitals were accredited by the Joint Commission on Accreditation of Hospitals in 1958, and all were members of the American Hospital Association. None of the hospitals belonged to state and/or regional hospital associations.

Of necessity, naval hospitals are located in areas where large contingents of naval forces are based in ports from which such forces operate. In 1958 most of the continental hospitals were in cities on the

Atlantic, Pacific, and Gulf Coasts. The three overseas hospitals were in Cuba, Guam, and Japan.

Financial data. In the 1957 fiscal year naval hospitals expended more than $110 million, of which nearly $77,800,000 was for inpatient care. Payroll expenses in the same period approximated $58,800,000.

The above operating costs reflect a number of expenses not normally incurred in nonmilitary hospitals, such as the pay and allowances granted to physicians and to personnel performing nonhospital functions.

The total capital invested in naval hospitals was almost $223 million, or about $14,000 per bed.

Naval hospitals are supported by Congressional appropriations and by income received from the Army and Air Force for occasional medical services rendered to their personnel. Capital funds are also appropriated by Congress.

Education and Research Activities. Nine naval hospitals were approved by the American Medical Association for residency training in 1957, and fourteen were approved for internships. Five naval hospitals were approved by the Bureau of Medicine and Surgery for affiliation with civilian hospitals and medical schools. Some of these were informal affiliations for the benefit of naval residency training only.

None of the naval hospitals operated professional nursing schools. However, a limited number of female enlisted personnel were being sponsored by the Navy in professional nursing courses at various colleges and universities.

While none of the hospitals operated practical nursing schools, the Navy was maintaining an excellent Hospital Corps School. Enlisted personnel graduating from this school serve in about the same capacity as a licensed practical nurse and appear to be as well qualified as graduates of approved schools of practical nursing.

In addition to the above, the Navy maintains specialized schools and training courses for medical officers in field and amphibious, aviation, submarine, atomic, and preventive medicine. Naval hospitals also provide technical training courses for enlisted personnel in such paramedical fields as laboratory, X-ray, pharmacy, chemistry, dentistry, and many others.

Research also plays an important role in the medical program of the Navy. The Navy Medical Research Institute in Bethesda, Maryland, is conducting a number of investigations on the medical aspects of naval service. In addition, there are a number of research laboratories in the United States and overseas which are under the management or technical control of the Bureau of Medicine and Surgery.

Administration. Naval hospitals are commanded by Medical Corps

Figure 8. Organization Chart, United States Naval Hospital, 1956

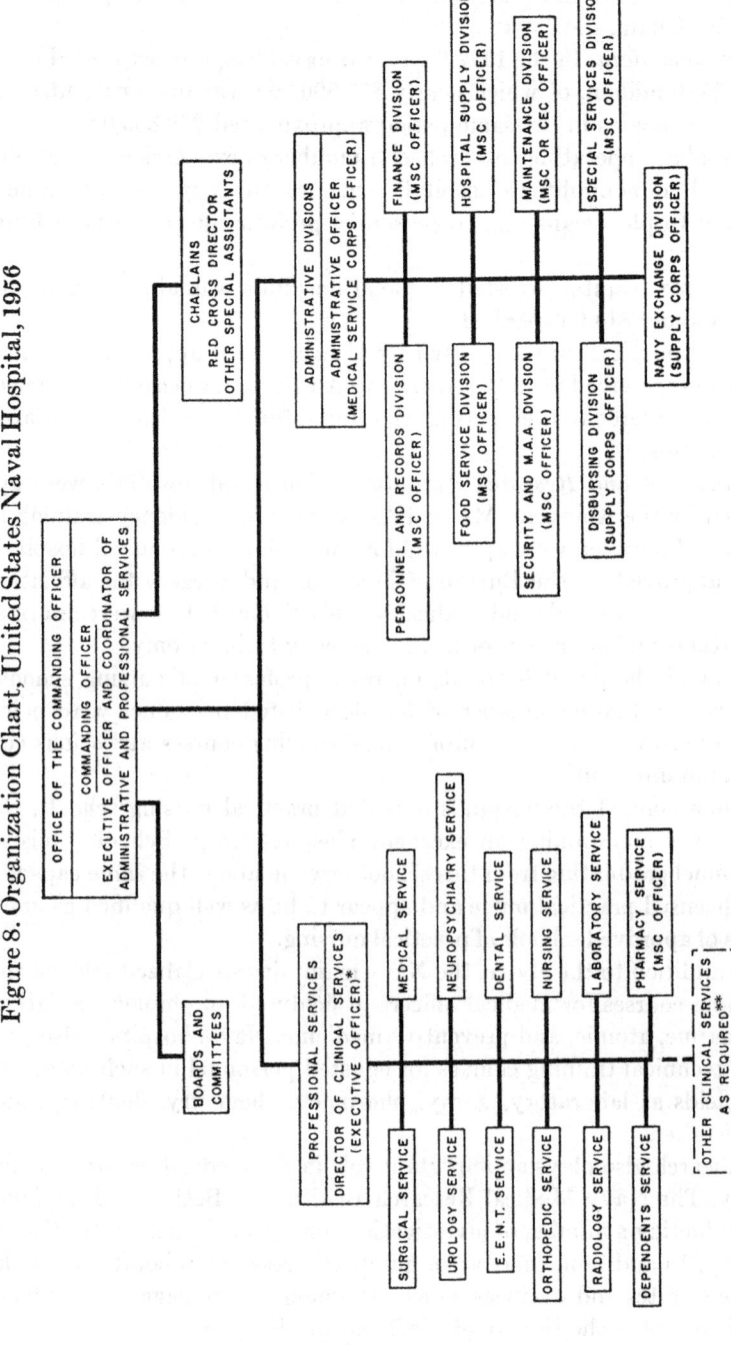

* The executive officer will also serve as chief of a clinical service in certain hospitals.
** A specialty may be organized as a service when it is headed by a board-certified specialist.

officers. They usually hold the rank of Captain and are responsible to the Surgeon General of the Navy for the operation of their institutions. The executive officer of a naval hospital is also a medical officer and is next in rank to the commanding officer.

A naval hospital is normally divided into administrative and professional services divisions (see Fig. 8). The latter division is usually headed by a Director of Clinical or Professional Services who, in certain hospitals, may also be the executive officer of the institution. The administrative division is directed by an officer of the Medical Service Corps.

Medical Staff. The medical staff of a naval hospital is organized by clinical services under the Director of Clinical or Professional Services. Appointments to the Medical Corps, promotions, and duty assignments are made by the Bureau of Naval Personnel on the recommendations of the Bureau of Medicine and Surgery.

Trends. The Navy is in the process of modernizing its hospital facilities and, on a planned long-range basis, is replacing obsolete and outdated temporary structures with permanent facilities of the latest design. Unless war breaks out, however, the total number of naval hospitals and beds should remain fairly stable.

UNITED STATES AIR FORCE HOSPITALS

The primary mission of the Air Force Medical Service is "to provide the medical support needed to maintain the highest possible degree of combat readiness and effectiveness in the Air Force." To accomplish this mission, the Air Force operates a large number of hospitals, dispensaries, and other medical facilities within the continental limits of the United States and overseas.

Organizational Structure and Governing Authority. The Department of the Air Force functions as part of the Department of Defense and is under the general direction and control of the President of the United States and the Secretary of Defense. The Secretary of the Air Force exercises immediate control over the department and is responsible for the conduct of all Air Force affairs (see Fig. 9).

The Chief of Staff, United States Air Force, under the direction of the Secretary of the Air Force, supervises all elements and personnel of the United States Air Force and exercises command over the Air Defense Command, the Strategic Air Command, and the Tactical Air Command.

The Surgeon General of the Air Force is the medical staff advisor to the Secretary of the Air Force and to the Chief of Staff. He supervises the Air Force Medical Service and reports directly to the Chief of Staff. The Surgeon General, however, does not have line authority over the

41

Figure 9. Department of the Air Force, 1956

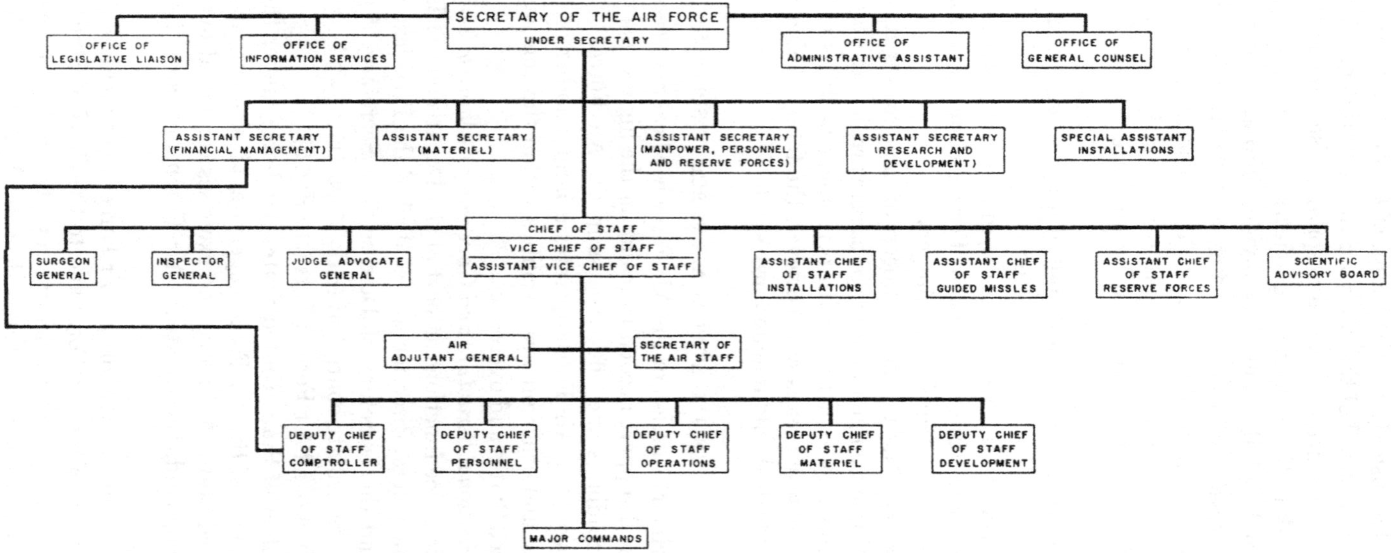

42

individual Air Force hospitals and dispensaries. These facilities are the responsibility of the commanders of the major air commands and the component base commands in which they are located.

Admission Requirements. Statutory authority and Air Force regulations govern the hospitalization of all Air Force personnel and of all other persons authorized to receive care under certain circumstances and conditions. Hospital and medical care is provided on the approval of the commanders of the various facilities. They may furnish care to authorized patients who are *not* uniformed service personnel if space, facilities, and staff are available.

History of Growth and Development. The National Security Act of 1947, which established the Department of the Air Force and made it a part of the Department of Defense, authorized the Secretary of Defense to transfer functions together with personnel, property, records, installations, agencies, and activities from the Army to the Air Force within a period of two years. On May 12, 1949, Secretary of Defense Louis Johnson accordingly directed the Air Force to assume responsibility for its own medical support and on July 1, 1949, the United States Air Force Medical Service came into being.

From the standpoint of physical facilities, the Medical Service was poorly prepared in the beginning to carry out its medical mission. Permanent hospital facilities were almost totally lacking and temporary facilities, constructed for the most part during World War II, were poorly maintained and were so inadequate in some cases that it was necessary to limit the scope of professional activity. To alleviate these shortcomings, the Air Force initiated an expansion and improvement program that made extraordinary progress in the period from 1949 to 1958. In July of 1949, only seventy-eight medical facilities were in operation with a capacity of 7050 beds. By 1958 the Air Force was maintaining 270 hospitals and dispensaries with a combined capacity of nearly 13,000 beds.

Measures of Significance. The Air Force feels the effectiveness of a squadron of jet fighters is impaired to a much greater degree by the illness and/or hospitalization of half a dozen pilots, mechanics, or other skilled personnel than an Army infantry company or naval vessel losing the same number of men through similar circumstances. For this reason, the Air Force considers it necessary to maintain a hospital or dispensary at almost every Air Force installation to provide the preventive and curative medical and hospital care necessary to keep the number of hospitalizations and the length of patient stay at an absolute minimum.

As a result of this philosophy, the Department of the Air Force operates a large number of relatively small hospitals and dispensaries. These facilities are scattered throughout the United States and are widely dispersed overseas. At the end of 1958 the Air Force maintained 137 hospitals, sixty-eight "Class A" dispensaries with bed accommodations and sixty-five "Class B" dispensaries without bed accommodations. Ninety-four hospitals and thirty-four "Class A" dispensaries were within the continental limits of the United States. Forty-three hospitals and thirty-four of the bed dispensaries were overseas.

The total capacity of all the hospital and dispensary facilities was 12,712 operating beds. Approximately 93 per cent of these beds were in hospitals. Nearly 75 per cent were in hospitals and dispensaries in the United States. During 1958 almost 450,000 patients were admitted to these beds, or about 35 admissions per bed. The average daily census was 9571 patients and the average occupancy rate was about 75 per cent.

As of May 1958, only 23 per cent of the Air Force hospitals had 100 or more beds and the average capacity was 86 beds. The continental hospitals ranged in size from four 25-bed installations in Indiana, Nebraska, Oklahoma, and Texas to the 980-bed institution at Lackland Air Force Base in San Antonio, Texas. Overseas, they ranged from a 15-bed hospital at Sevilla Air Base in Spain to a 320-bed installation in Wiesbaden, Germany. The largest "Class A" dispensaries contained only 24 beds and the average capacity was under 12 beds.

At the beginning of 1958, forty-six hospitals — roughly 34 per cent of the total number maintained — were accredited by the Joint Commission on Accreditation of Hospitals. Forty-two of these hospitals were in the United States and four were overseas. Twenty-nine hospitals were members of the American Hospital Association.

Approximately 40,600 persons were employed in Air Force hospitals and "Class A" and "Class B" dispensaries in the latter part of 1958, including almost 8000 civilian employees. An additional 8000 military and civilian personnel were engaged in medical activities not directly connected with hospitals or dispensaries.

Figure 10. Air Force Medical Treatment Facility, 1956

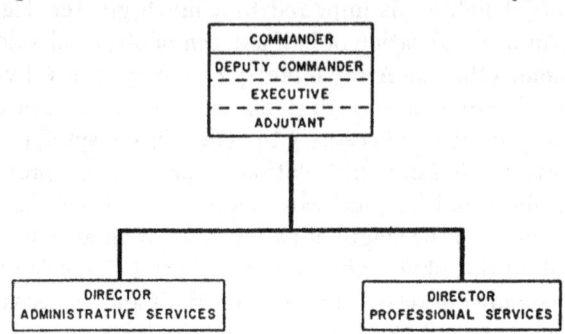

Financial Data. The total cost of operating the hospitals and "Class A" dispensaries in the 1957 fiscal year was nearly $153 million. Payroll expenses exceeded $114,500,000 and the payroll component of total expenses, including full-time physicians, approximated 74 per cent.

In the same year, Air Force hospitals, dispensaries, dental clinics, and other medical buildings had an estimated value of nearly $204 million. Medical facilities under construction at that time represented an additional investment of close to $98 million.

Congressional appropriations are the primary source of both operating income and capital funds.

Educational Activities. Only one Air Force hospital had been approved by the American Medical Association for internships in 1958 and four were approved for residency training. One hospital was affiliated with a medical school. None of the hospitals operated either a professional or practical nursing school.

In the early part of 1958 the Department of the Air Force reported 719 officers were in training in Air Force, Army, and civilian hospitals. Included in the total were medical and dental interns, medical residents, and hospital administration residents and students. In addition, 1243 enlisted personnel were receiving medical technician training in schools operated by the Air Force, Army, and Navy.

Administration. The command element of an Air Force hospital normally consists of a hospital commander, a deputy commander, an executive officer, and an adjutant (see Fig. 10). The hospital commander is always a Medical Corps officer and is usually the senior medical officer on the base in which the hospital is located. He administers and super-

Figure 11. Administrative Services Division, Air Force Hospital, 1956

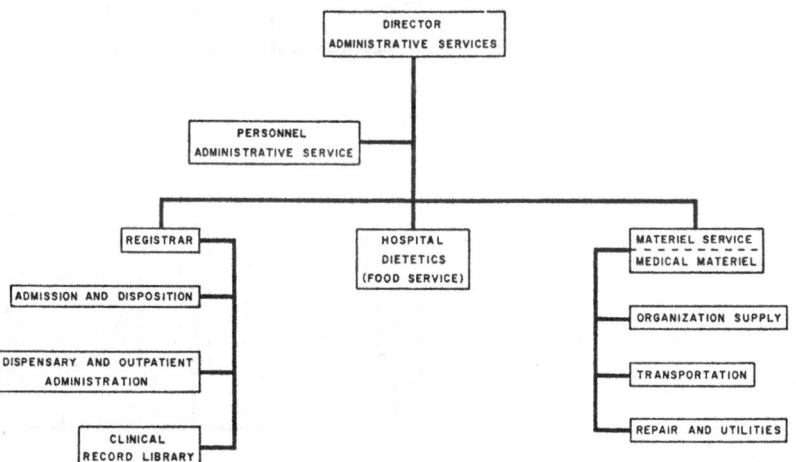

Figure 12. Professional Services Division, Air Force Hospital, 1956

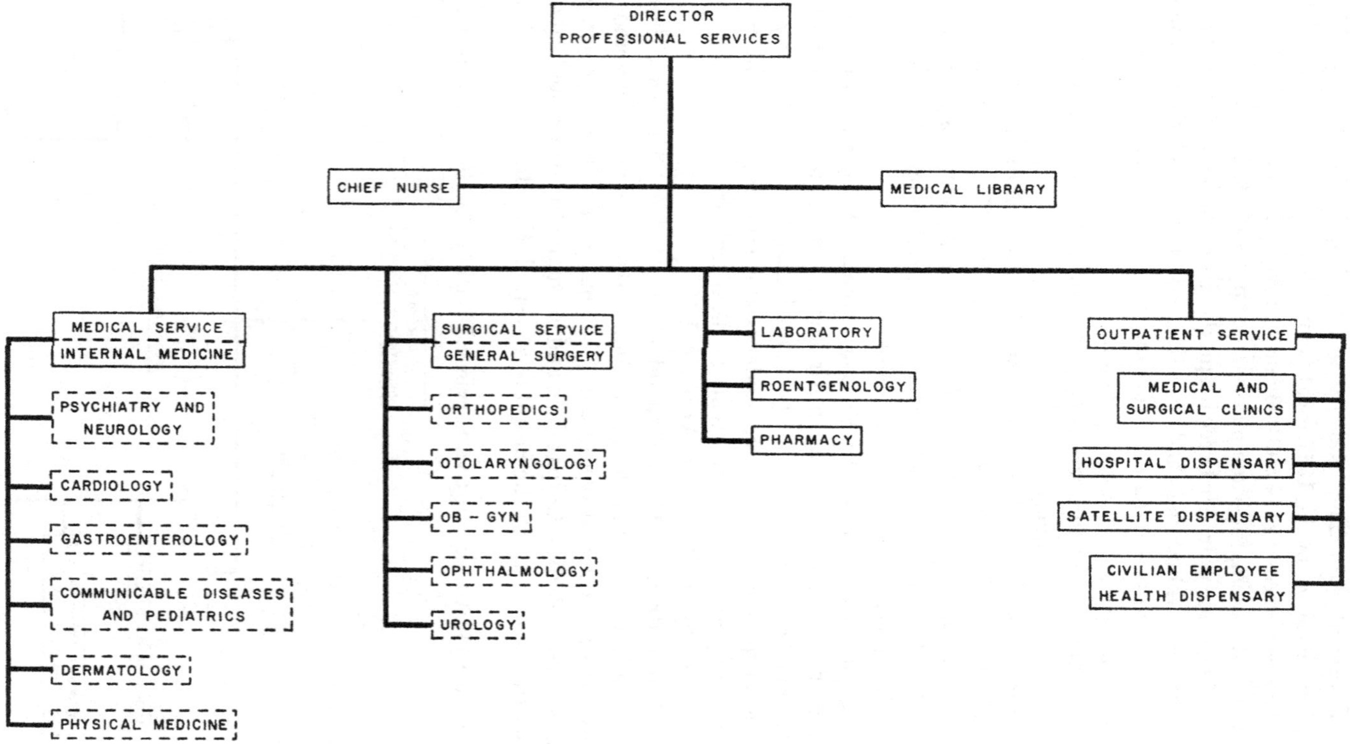

DIRECTOR
PROFESSIONAL SERVICES

MEDICAL LIBRARY

CHIEF NURSE

MEDICAL SERVICE
INTERNAL MEDICINE

PSYCHIATRY AND
NEUROLOGY

CARDIOLOGY

GASTROENTEROLOGY

COMMUNICABLE DISEASES
AND PEDIATRICS

DERMATOLOGY

PHYSICAL MEDICINE

SURGICAL SERVICE
GENERAL SURGERY

ORTHOPEDICS

OTOLARYNGOLOGY

OB - GYN

OPHTHALMOLOGY

UROLOGY

LABORATORY

ROENTGENOLOGY

PHARMACY

OUTPATIENT SERVICE

MEDICAL AND
SURGICAL CLINICS

HOSPITAL DISPENSARY

SATELLITE DISPENSARY

CIVILIAN EMPLOYEE
HEALTH DISPENSARY

vises the hospital and is directly responsible to the base commander for hospital operation. The executive officer functions primarily as an administrative assistant to the hospital commander and belongs to the Medical Service Corps.

Air Force hospitals are divided into professional services and administrative services (see Figs. 11 and 12). Each of these divisions is headed by a director who serves as an assistant to the hospital commander and who is responsible directly to him.

The internal organization and functional structure of an Air Force hospital varies with the size of the institution and with local conditions. Some large hospitals require, in addition to the hospital commander and the adjutant, a deputy hospital commander and an executive officer in the command element. Hospital commanders frequently assume other duties. Usually, they act as base surgeons and, on occasion, may serve as base medical inspectors and/or base veterinarians. In some hospitals, one officer may function both as the director of administrative services and as the executive officer.

Medical Staff. To be eligible for an appointment as a medical officer in the Air Force, a physician must (1) possess a degree of doctor of medicine from a school of medicine which is acceptable to the Surgeon General of the Air Force; (2) have completed one year of internship and be engaged in the ethical practice of medicine; (3) possess a license to practice medicine in a state or territory of the United States or in the District of Columbia or possess a diploma from the National Board of Medical Examiners.

Qualified physicians are normally given the rank of first lieutenant. However, they may be appointed to higher grades if they possess professional experience and education which exceeds that required above.

The medical staff of an Air Force hospital is organized by clinical services under a Director of Professional Services.

Trends. The future development of the Air Force Medical Service, including hospital expansion, naturally is contingent on the development of the Air Force itself in the coming years. Hospital planning is currently centered on the construction of hospitals and dispensaries at bases and locations which, at present, do not have such facilities and on the replacement of existing, obsolete hospitals with permanent structures.

VETERANS ADMINISTRATION HOSPITALS

The Veterans Administration (VA), an independent agency of the executive branch of the federal government, administers benefits authorized by law for veterans and the dependents of deceased veterans.

The major purposes of the VA may be grouped as follows:

Patterns of Hospital Ownership and Control

1. To provide medical care and treatment for eligible beneficiaries.

2. To afford financial assistance to veterans and their families; to compensate veterans for loss of earning power because of disabilities incurred in service in the Armed Forces; and to aid them in their rehabilitation and readjustment to normal civilian pursuits.

3. To administer a program of life insurance for certain servicemen and veterans as authorized by Congress.

Organization Structure and Governing Authority. To carry out the above purposes, three basic operating departments have been established: the Department of Medicine and Surgery, the Department of Veterans Benefits, and the Department of Insurance (see Fig. 13). Assisting the three basic departments are staff offices which plan and evaluate the various programs and provide the supporting administrative services.

The Administrator of Veterans Affairs is responsible for the operation

Figure 13. Organization of the Veterans Administration, 1956

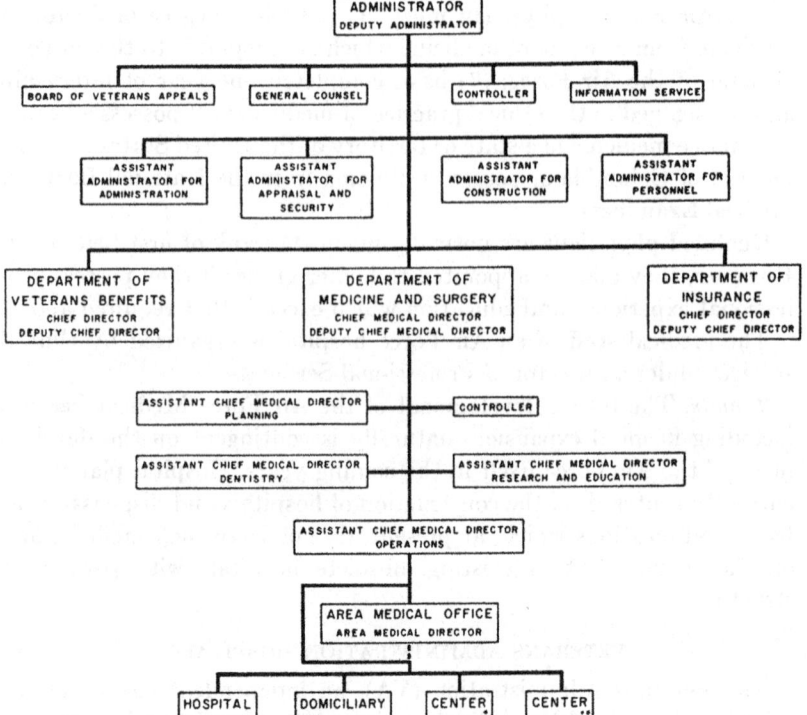

* Hospital and domiciliary center combined.
** Hospital and regional office combined.

of the VA. He is appointed by the President and serves as the President's advisor on veterans' affairs.

The Chief Medical Director is responsible for the activities of the Department of Medicine and Surgery. He is aided by a deputy and four assistant chief medical directors, a controller, and seven area medical offices.

The area medical offices have limited supervisory authority and serve primarily in an advisory capacity.

Persons Eligible for Care in Veterans Administration Hospitals. The Veterans Administration is charged by law and regulation with the responsibility of providing hospital care to four separate groups of patients:

1. Those requiring treatment for service-connected disabilities. This group is unconditionally eligible for care and it is the policy of the VA to offer immediate hospitalization to veterans in this category. On November 30, 1956, a census revealed 35 per cent of the total number of patients receiving care in VA hospitals were being treated for service-connected conditions.

2. Those requiring treatment for non-service-connected conditions who were either discharged from military service for a disability incurred or aggravated in line of duty or who have a compensable service-connected disability. This group is eligible for care if beds are available and, on the above date, 8.6 per cent of the VA hospital patients were in this classification.

3. Other veterans with wartime service who require treatment for non-service-connected conditions. This group is eligible for treatment if beds are available and if they are not able to pay for private hospital care. Such patients must indicate on an affidavit that they are unable to defray the cost of hospitalization and must support this affidavit with a statement of assets. On November 30, 1956, 55.4 per cent of the VA patient load fell into this category.

4. Nonveterans with specific entitlement. This group consists primarily of military personnel who have been transferred into VA hospitals from military installations and who are in the process of being separated from the armed services to continue treatment for their service-connected disabilities in VA hospitals. They are classified as "nonveterans" until they are actually separated from military service. Less than one per cent of the patients hospitalized on November 30, 1956 were in this group.

History of Growth and Development of Veterans' Benefits and Veterans' Medical Care. The first recorded law in America affording benefits to veterans was enacted in 1636 by the Pilgrims of Plymouth Colony while they were at war with the Pequod Indians. This law provided that "if any man shalbee sent forth as a souldier and shall return maimed, hee shalbee maintained competently by the Collonie during his life."

The other colonies followed suit with similar laws, and by the time the colonies were welded together as a single nation, the concept of benefits for veterans was well established. As one of its first acts, the Continental Congress in 1776 sought to encourage enlistments and curtail desertions by passing a nation-wide law providing for the care of men disabled while serving in the armed forces. This act, as did earlier laws dealing with benefits to veterans, placed the primary emphasis on pensions.

The first domiciliary and medical facility for veterans was provided by the federal government in 1811 with the establishment of the U.S. Naval Home in Philadelphia as a "permanent home for disabled and decrepit officers, seamen, and mariners." The first federal homes for disabled and invalid soldiers were authorized by Congress in 1851.

In 1861 the Secretary of War appointed a Sanitary Commission to study the medical and hospital problems of the Union Armies. The Commission found it was necessary to give "special relief" to needy and sick soldiers who had been discharged from military service because of wounds and disabilities and for whom Army regulations failed to provide necessary care. Consequently, the Commission recommended a medical program affording temporary care to such soldiers in hospitals and domiciliaries in various parts of the country. This led to the establishment by Congress, at the end of the Civil War, of the National Asylum for Disabled Volunteer Soldiers — in reality, a number of homes scattered throughout the nation.

The veteran population has increased with each subsequent war and facilities to serve these veterans have been greatly expanded. The most startling growth in VA hospitals and domiciliaries occurred in the decade from 1946 to 1956. With the end of World War II, some nineteen million servicemen suddenly became potential VA beneficiaries and a gigantic expansion of VA facilities became paramount. As a result, old hospitals were modernized and enlarged and many new hospitals were established. The total number of operating beds in VA hospitals increased by 25 per cent during the period.

History of Growth and Development of the Veterans Administration. The Veterans Administration, as we know it today, is a consolidation of three agencies which formerly handled veterans' affairs. It was established in 1930 and took over the functions of the Pension Bureau, the National Home for Disabled Volunteer Soldiers and the Veterans Bureau.

In 1819 Congress gave up all control over veterans' pensions and the Secretary of War was given full power to administer the pension program. Actual administration was carried on by the War Department's Bureau of Pensions. In 1849 this bureau was transferred by the War Department into the newly-created Department of Interior where it remained until its consolidation as the Veterans Administration.

As discussed previously, the National Asylum for Disabled Volunteer Soldiers was formed in 1866 to provide domiciliary, hospital, and medical care in its individual homes or branches. In 1873 the word "Home" was substituted for "Asylum."

A commission was appointed by President Harding in 1921 to study the problem of administering veterans' benefits. As a result of the commission's recommendations, the United States Veterans Bureau was created in the same year. While this bureau was an improvement over the previous method of administering benefits, it did not solve all the problems that arise when responsibility is divided. Three agencies were still providing benefits independently, causing delays and increasing the amount of necessary paperwork.

Consolidation of the three agencies into a single organization was suggested to Congress by President Hoover in his State of the Union message in 1929. Congress reacted to this proposal the following year by creating the Veterans Administration.

Measures of Significance. At the end of the 1958 fiscal year, the Veterans Administration was maintaining 172 hospitals including 112 general medical and surgical, forty psychiatric, and twenty tuberculosis institutions. Their combined capacity was 120,526 operating beds.

During that year, approximately 490,000 patients were admitted to VA hospitals, or slightly more than four admissions per bed. In addition, over 31,000 VA beneficiaries were admitted to hospitals not operated by the Veterans Administration.

The average daily census in the VA hospitals in that same period was just under 111,600 patients and the average occupancy rate exceeded 90 per cent.

Roughly 117,000 persons were employed in these hospitals during the year, or about 1.06 employees per patient. The Department of Medicine and Surgery appoints physicians, dentists, and nurses to positions in VA hospitals. All other employees, including the administrative staffs, pharmacists, dietitians, and nonprofessional personnel, are appointed under the rules and regulations of the United States Civil Service Commission.

At the end of the 1958 fiscal year, the VA hospitals ranged in size from the 56-bed general medical and surgical hospital in Bonham, Texas, to the 3621-bed medical center in Los Angeles. Approximately 49 per cent of the hospitals had a rated capacity of more than 500 beds and the average operating capacity was 701 beds.

Geographically, the VA hospitals are well distributed. Every state in the Union had at least one such institution in 1958 and none of the American Hospital Association regions contained less than twelve or more than twenty-five VA hospitals. Veteran population is the primary basis for the distribution of these institutions.

The Joint Commission on Accreditation of Hospitals had accredited 169, or about 98 per cent, of the VA hospitals at the end of the above fiscal year. All of the hospitals were members of the American Hospital Association and most of them were associated with state and regional hospital organizations.

Financial Data. The hospitals operated by the Veterans Administration expended approximately $661 million during the 1958 fiscal year. An additional $13–14 million was expended in caring for VA beneficiaries in non-VA hospitals.

The payroll component of total expenses approximated 80 per cent, which was much higher than the national average for all hospitals. However, it must be pointed out that the VA hospital expenses include salaries paid physicians and dentists that are normally not incorporated in the expenditures of other hospitals.

Total assets of the 172 VA hospitals were estimated to be $1,218,-540,000, or slightly over $10,100 per bed.

Federal tax revenues are the primary source of both operating income and capital funds and the United States Congress appropriates the money required for these purposes.

Educational and Research Activities. The Veterans Administration feels that patient care is optimal and the professional environment is more stimulating in hospitals which conduct teaching and research programs. Consequently, in its desire to provide its beneficiaries with medical and hospital care that is "second to none," the VA has greatly increased its educational and research activities in the past decade.

Over 54 per cent of the VA hospitals were approved for residencies by the American Medical Association in 1958, 4 per cent were approved for internships, and 47 per cent maintained affiliations with medical schools. The total number of students in the various educational programs in April of 1958 included 2015 medical residents, 29 dental residents, 76 medical interns, and 22 dental interns. In addition, nearly 5000 medical students were serving as clinical clerks.

None of the hospitals operated either professional or practical nursing schools. However, twenty-nine VA hospitals were providing affiliate experience of from six to twelve weeks for professional nursing students.

The medical research program of the Veterans Administration em-

Figure 14. Organization Chart, Veterans Administration Hospital, 1956

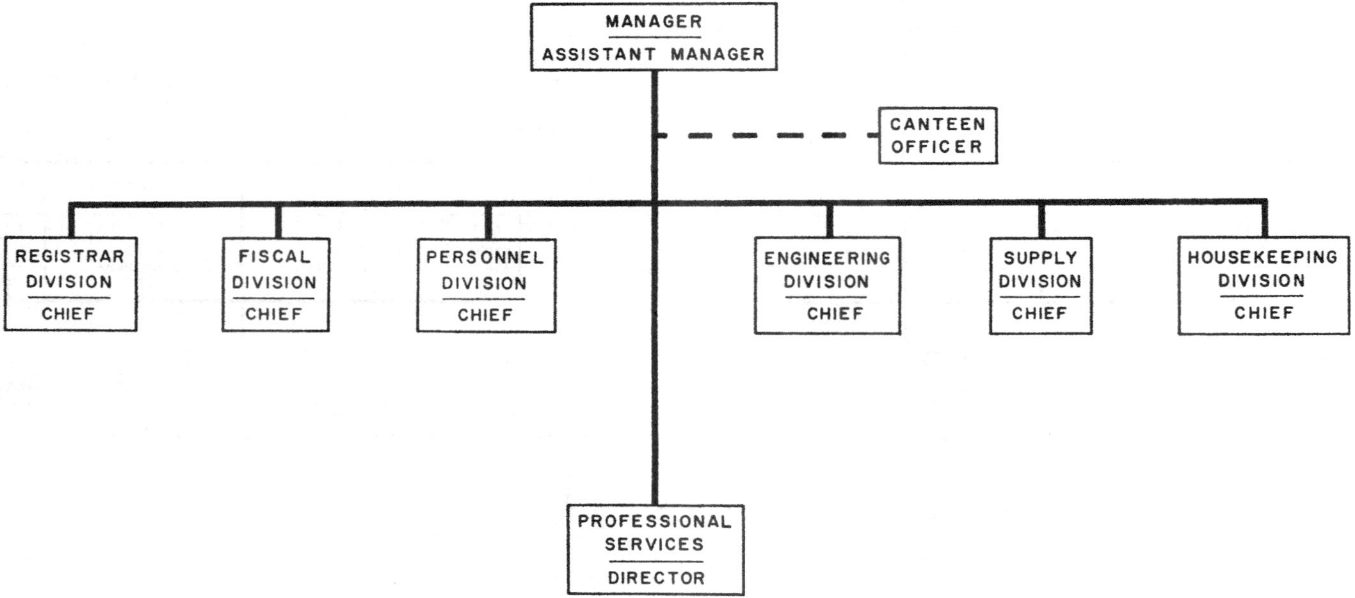

MANAGER
ASSISTANT MANAGER

CANTEEN OFFICER

REGISTRAR DIVISION
CHIEF

FISCAL DIVISION
CHIEF

PERSONNEL DIVISION
CHIEF

ENGINEERING DIVISION
CHIEF

SUPPLY DIVISION
CHIEF

HOUSEKEEPING DIVISION
CHIEF

PROFESSIONAL SERVICES
DIRECTOR

Figure 15. Organization Chart, Veterans Administration Regional Office–Hospital Center, 1956

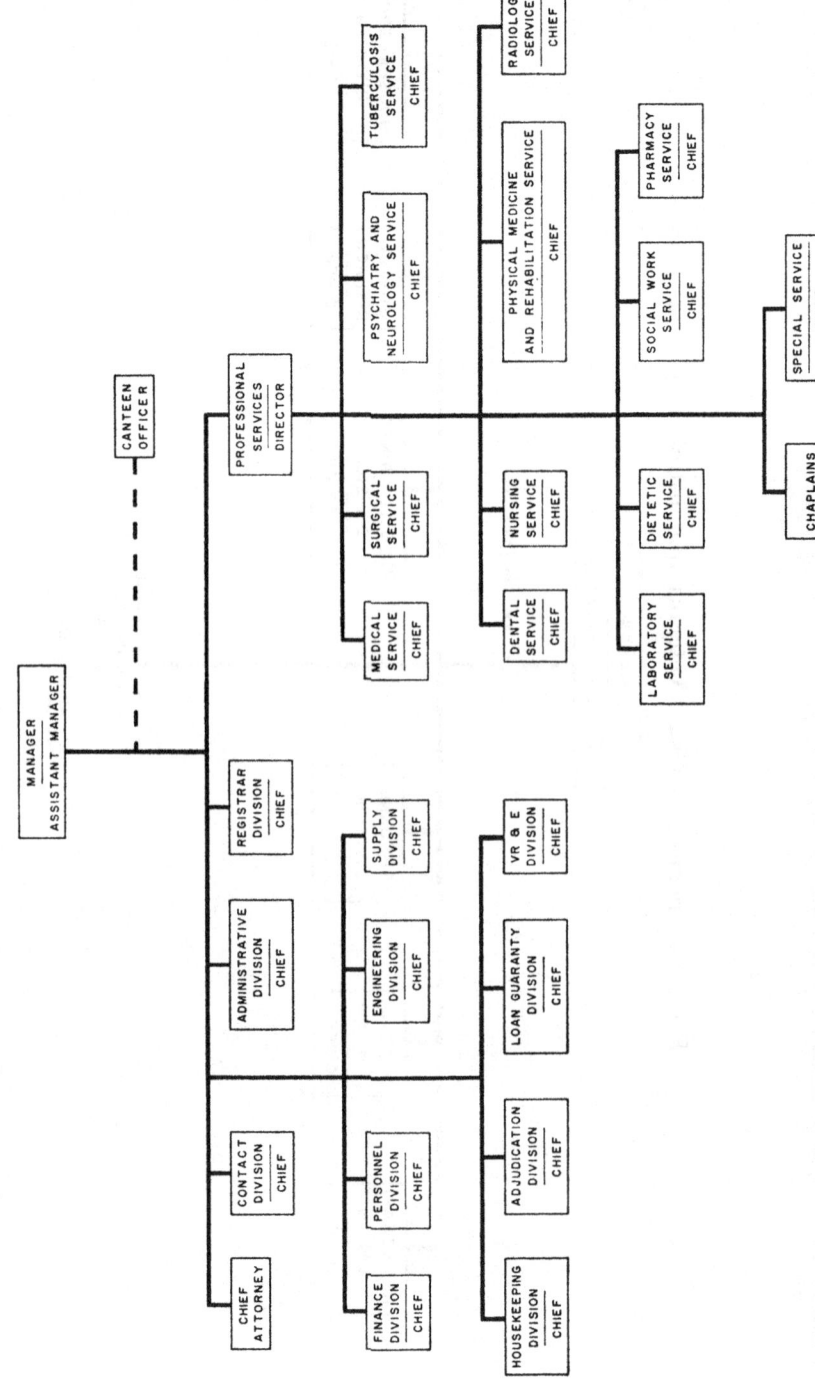

phasizes studies of the major health problems of the veteran population. Recently, this has been reflected in a significant increase in the number of research projects dealing with heart disease, cancer, nervous and mental diseases, tuberculosis, and the problems of the aging. In a number of instances, research projects are being conducted on a cooperative basis by staff members of several VA hospitals.

Administration. Managers of VA hospitals are appointed by the chief executive of the Veterans Administration — the Administrator of Veterans Affairs — after a selection committee has submitted its recommendations. In the past, most hospital managers were traditionally members of the medical profession. At present, however, a substantial number of managers of VA hospitals are nonmedical people. This is particularly true where hospitals have been combined with regional offices or domiciliaries.

Figure 16. Organization Chart, Veterans Administration
Hospital–Domiciliary Center

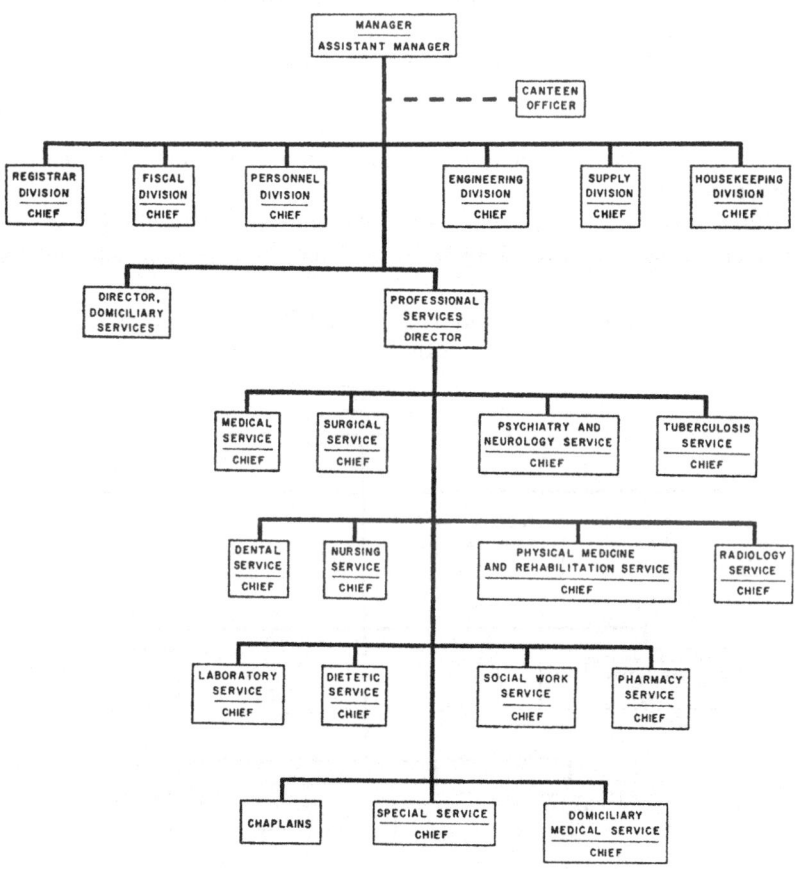

Patterns of Hospital Ownership and Control

Administrative control over the individual hospitals is exercised by the Chief Medical Director within the framework of Congressional mandates and under the direction of general policies laid down by the Administrator of Veterans Affairs. Hospital managers are responsible for the operation of their institutions to the Chief Medical Director and he, in turn, is responsible to the Administrator of Veterans Affairs. Where hospitals are combined with regional offices, the managers are responsible to the Chief Medical Director for medical activities and to the Chief Benefits Director for regional office activities.

The Director of Professional Services in each hospital directs and coordinates the professional services of the hospital for the manager. The manager may designate either the Director of Professional Services, or the assistant manager to act for him in his absence. Organization of the single hospital, of the hospital combined with a regional office, and of the hospital combined with a domiciliary center are shown in Figures 14, 15, and 16.

Medical Staff. To be eligible for appointment to a position in a VA hospital, a physician must (1) be a citizen of the United States; (2) hold a degree of Doctor of Medicine or Osteopathy from an approved college or university; (3) have completed a one-year internship in an approved hospital; (4) be licensed to practice medicine, surgery, or osteopathy in one of the states or territories of the United States or in the District of Columbia.

Physicians who are appointed to full-time positions are salaried employees of the Veterans Administration. Salaries are commensurate with

Figure 17. Professional Services Division, Veterans
Administration Hospital, 1956

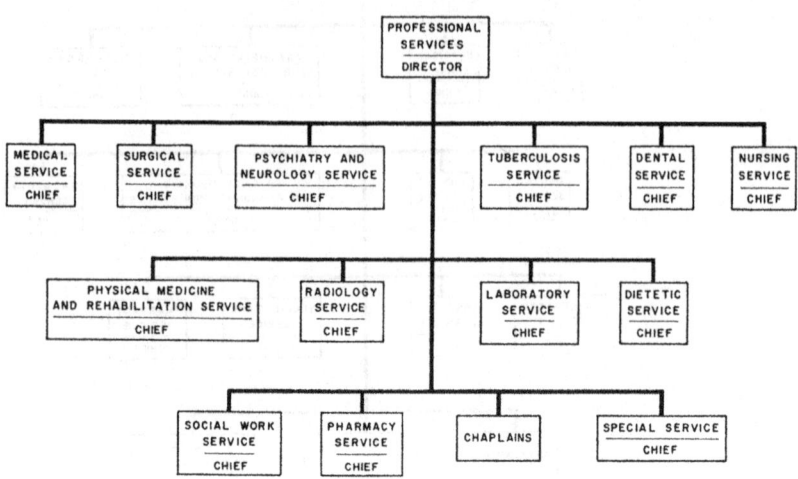

the number of years of practice and the professional attainments that have been acquired.

The professional program in a VA hospital is directed and coordinated by the Director of Professional Services (see Fig. 17). The medical staff is divided into major or clinical services, each with its own chief, in a manner similar to most civilian general-acute hospitals of corresponding size.

Trends. As the veteran population from the recent wars becomes older, it will require a proportionately greater amount of medical care. The extent to which the VA should assume any increased responsibility for providing that care for non-service-connected disabilities involves a question of national policy. As a result, the future expansion of VA hospital facilities is impossible to accurately determine.

Upon completion of the *presently* authorized building and modernization program, the Veterans Administration will have 171 hospitals with an ultimate rated capacity of 126,000 beds. However, a continuation of the current decline in tuberculosis patients may warrant the closing of some of the tuberculosis hospitals.

THE DEPARTMENT OF HEALTH, EDUCATION, AND WELFARE AND THE UNITED STATES PUBLIC HEALTH SERVICE

The Department of Health, Education, and Welfare was created in 1953 under a reorganization plan which abolished the Federal Security Agency and transferred all functions of the Federal Security Administrator to the Secretary of Health, Education, and Welfare. As its name implies, the department is responsible for promoting the general welfare in the fields of health, education, and social security (see Fig. 18). In carrying out these responsibilities, the department operates a number of hospitals and medical facilities in the United States and its territorial possessions. All of these institutions, with the exception of Saint Elizabeth's Hospital in Washington, D.C., are administered by the Public Health Service, an operating agency of the department.

The Secretary of Health, Education, and Welfare supervises and directs departmental operations and, as head of an executive department of the federal government, reports directly to the President of the United States. The Under Secretary assists the Secretary in the administration of all department agencies and is primarily responsible for the department's organization and management activities. The department maintains nine regional offices, and the regional directors represent the Secretary, carry out department policies, and provide leadership, coordination, evaluation, and general administrative supervision within their respective regions.

Figure 18. The Department of Health, Education, and Welfare, 1956

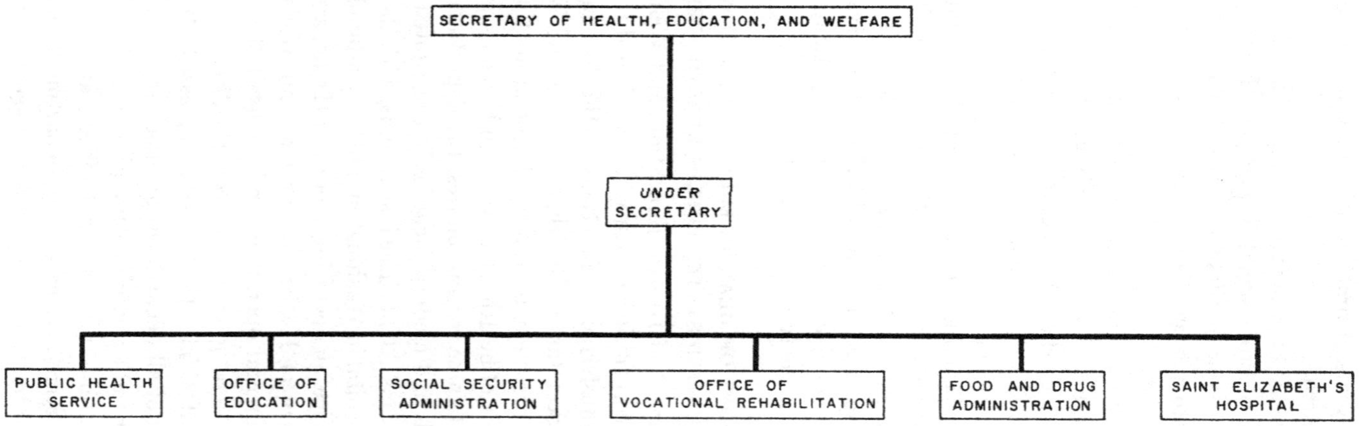

SECRETARY OF HEALTH, EDUCATION, AND WELFARE

UNDER SECRETARY

PUBLIC HEALTH SERVICE

OFFICE OF EDUCATION

SOCIAL SECURITY ADMINISTRATION

OFFICE OF VOCATIONAL REHABILITATION

FOOD AND DRUG ADMINISTRATION

SAINT ELIZABETH'S HOSPITAL

The United States Public Health Service. The Public Health Service is the federal agency which is specifically responsible for protecting and improving the health of the people of the United States. Its major functions are (1) to conduct and support research and training in the medical and related sciences and in public health methods and administration; (2) to assist state and local governments in the application of new knowledge for the prevention and control of disease, the maintenance of a healthful environment, and the development of community health services; (3) to provide medical and hospital services to persons authorized to receive care from the Public Health Service, to aid in the development of the nation's hospitals and related facilities, and to prevent the introduction of communicable diseases into the United States and its possessions.

Organizational Structure and Governing Authority. To carry out the above functions, the activities of the Service have been organized into three operating bureaus: the National Institutes of Health, the Bureau of State Services, and the Bureau of Medical Services (see Fig. 19). A fourth bureau, the Office of the Surgeon General, consists primarily of staff services for the three operating bureaus and the Surgeon General.

The Surgeon General is a commissioned officer in the Public Health Service appointed by the President for a four-year term. He is responsible to the Secretary of Health, Education, and Welfare for the activities of the Service and is assisted in planning, coordinating, and administering these activities by the chiefs of the three operating bureaus, by various staff offices, and by the National Advisory Health Council and other special advisory groups, in the fields of cancer, heart disease, mental health, dental research, arthritis, and metabolic diseases, neurology and blindness, hospital planning and construction, and

Figure 19. The United States Public Health Service, 1956

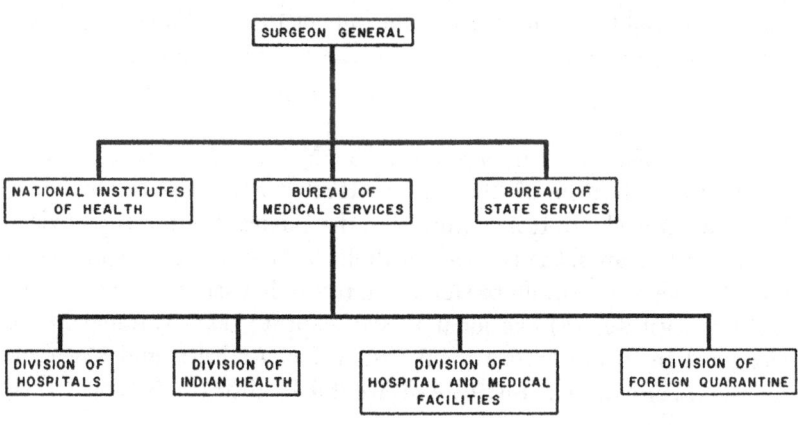

water pollution control. In addition, the Public Health Service maintains a staff in eight of the nine regional offices of the Department of Health, Education, and Welfare who represent the Surgeon General in interpreting and carrying out the broad general policies of the Service.

The Bureau of Medical Services. The Bureau of Medical Services is responsible for operating all Public Health Service hospitals except the Clinical Center of the National Institutes of Health. Through two of its divisions — the Division of Hospitals and the Division of Indian Health — the bureau provides hospitalization and medical care to the following groups: (1) American merchant seamen; (2) personnel of the United States Coast Guard and the Coast and Geodetic Survey and their dependents; (3) Public Health Service commissioned officers and their dependents; (4) American Indians and Alaskan natives; (5) federal employees injured on duty; (6) persons with leprosy; (7) persons who are addicted to narcotic drugs; (8) active duty officers and enlisted personnel of the armed services and their dependents under the terms of the Dependents' Medical Care Act.

In addition, the bureau supervises Freedmen's Hospital in Washington, D.C. This is a general-acute institution, principally concerned with the treatment of Negro patients, which has an extensive system of specialized clinics for outpatients and which provides internships and clinical experience for graduates and students of the Negro medical school at Howard University.

The bureau also assigns Public Health Service medical and dental personnel to the ships and shore establishments of the United States Coast Guard and the Maritime Administration, to the prisons and reformatories of the Department of Justice, and to several other federal agencies.

Another division of the bureau, the Division of Hospital and Medical Facilities, administers the Hospital Survey and Construction Act (commonly referred to as the Hill-Burton Act) of 1946 and its amendments. The division approves state plans for the construction of hospital and related facilities and provides financial assistance to approved construction projects.

The National Institutes of Health. The National Institutes of Health — the research arm of the Public Health Service — is located at Bethesda, Maryland. It is composed of the Clinical Center, the Division of Research Grants, the Division of Biologics Standards, supporting administrative services, and the following research institutes: (1) National Cancer Institute; (2) National Heart Institute; (3) National Microbiological Institute; (4) National Institute of Arthritis and Metabolic Diseases; (5) National Institute of Mental Health; (6) National Institute of Neurological Diseases and Blindness; (7) National Institute of Dental Research.

Organizationally, the National Institutes of Health is a separate bureau of the Service. It is headed by an Assistant Surgeon General who reports directly to the Surgeon General of the Public Health Service.

History of Growth and Development. The history of the Public Health Service reflects specific events in the history of the United States. Originally called the United States Marine Hospital Service, it began in 1798 when an act of Congress providing "for the relief of sick and disabled seamen" was signed by President John Adams.

The number of hospitals operated by the Marine Hospital or Public Health Service has varied considerably from then until now. The first marine hospitals were established in Boston, Massachusetts, in 1799 and Norfolk, Virginia, in 1802. By 1861 twenty-seven such hospitals had been founded, more than one half of which were in cities located on interior lakes and rivers. At the turn of the century the Service was operating twenty-three hospitals, including a tuberculosis sanitarium. Following World War I, the Service was made responsible for the Bureau of War Risk Insurance beneficiaries and maintained eighty-one hospitals, including those of the War Department. With the establishment of the Veterans Bureau (now consolidated into the Veterans Administration) in 1921, the Service was relieved of the responsibility for these beneficiaries but continued to operate twenty-four hospitals. Also, in 1921, the Louisiana Leper Home was purchased by the federal government and assigned to the Public Health Service. The hospitals at Lexington, Kentucky, and Fort Worth, Texas, were opened in 1935 and 1938 respectively, primarily for the treatment of men and women addicted to narcotic drugs.

In 1955 responsibility for the operation of Indian hospitals and the Indian health program was transferred from the Interior Department's Bureau of Indian Affairs to the Public Health Service. Federal responsibility for Indian health dates back to the early 1800s. Probably the first contact Indians had with the "white man's medicine" was the occasional attention afforded them by Army medical officers on the early reservations. Some of the later treaties and agreements between various Indian tribes and the federal government provided that the latter would maintain a miller, a blacksmith, and a physician on certain reservations.

The first organized medical facilities for Indians were established in 1873. However, very few hospitals had been constructed at the turn of the century and nearly 90 per cent of the Indian institutions in operation in 1958 were founded in the period from 1910 to 1940. The first hospital for Alaskan natives was established in Juneau in 1916.

61

Patterns of Hospital Ownership and Control

Under the Public Health Service, Indian hospitals have centralized services, increased the number of personnel, and improved food service, maintenance, administration, and other functions.

Measures of Significance. In 1958 the Division of Hospitals of the Bureau of Medical Services was operating sixteen hospitals: twelve general-acute institutions, one tuberculosis hospital, a leprosarium, and two institutions for the treatment of narcotic addiction and other neuropsychiatric disorders — with a combined capacity of 6541 beds. The division was also maintaining twenty-five full-time outpatient clinics.

During 1957 the sixteen hospitals admitted nearly 49,000 patients, or a little more than seven admissions per bed. The average daily census was over 5300 patients and the average occupancy rate exceeded 80 per cent. The institutions employed approximately 5500 persons, or about one employee per patient.

Nine of the hospitals had over 300 beds in 1958 and the average capacity was nearly 409 beds. They ranged in size from a 140-bed general-acute institution in Memphis, Tennessee, to a 1264-bed neuropsychiatric hospital in Lexington, Kentucky.

Most of the hospitals were located along the coasts, waterways, and border areas of the United States. Six hospitals were on the eastern seaboard, two on the Gulf of Mexico, and two on the west coast. Six hospitals, including three of the four institutions offering specialized treatment, were located inland.

All sixteen hospitals were members of the American Hospital Association and their respective state and regional hospital associations in 1958. In addition, all were accredited by the Joint Commission on Accreditation of Hospitals.

The Division of Indian Health of the Bureau of Medical Services administers a comprehensive health and medical care program for some 340,000 American Indians and approximately 35,000 Alaskan Indians, Aleuts, and Eskimos. In 1958 the division operated fifty-five hospitals, including eight in Alaska, and contracted with more than 160 nonfederal institutions for hospital care for Indian patients.

In the same year, the fifty-five hospitals had a combined capacity of more than 3800 beds and admitted nearly 56,000 patients, or about 14 admissions per bed. The average daily census was about 2600 patients; the average occupancy rate was approximately 70 per cent.

Fifty-one of the fifty-five hospitals offered general-acute care. The remaining four were principally concerned with the treatment of tuberculosis.

Most of the Indian hospitals were quite small. Although they ranged in size from 15 to 400 beds, only nine hospitals had more than 100 beds and the average capacity was about 70 beds.

Approximately 3500 persons were employed in the fifty-five institutions, or roughly 1.3 employees per patient. Many of the employees were Indians and Alaskan natives who had been prepared for hospital positions in the division's schools of practical nursing and through on-the-job training programs.

Indian hospitals are located on reservations or in areas which have large Indian populations. Forty-six of the forty-eight Indian hospitals in the United States in 1958 were west of the Mississippi River. Of the American Hospital Association's geographic regions, the Mountain and West North Central regions contained the greatest number of these Indian institutions with twenty-two and thirteen hospitals respectively. Ten Indian hospitals — over 20 per cent of the total number in this country — were located in the State of Arizona.

Eleven of the fifty-five Indian hospitals were accredited by the Joint Commission on Accreditation of Hospitals. All were members of the American Hospital Association and a large proportion belonged to state and/or regional hospital associations.

The Clinical Center of the National Institutes of Health is a fourteen-story research facility which provides about twice as much space for laboratories as it does for patient care. In 1957 the center had 516 beds and admitted 2775 patients, or just over five admissions per bed. The average daily census was 321 patients and the average occupancy rate was roughly 62 per cent. The center employed 1485 persons during that year, or more than 4.6 employees per patient.

The center was accredited by the Joint Commission on Accreditation of Hospitals and was a member of the American Hospital Association and its respective state and regional associations.

Financial Data. The sixteen institutions operated by the Division of Hospitals expended nearly $32 million in 1957, or more than $16.00 per patient day. Payroll expenditures were about $24 million and the payroll component of total expenses was about 79 per cent. Total assets of these hospitals were estimated to exceed $54 million, or around $8200 per bed.

The Indian hospitals of the Division of Indian Health expended over $21 million in 1957, or roughly $21.00 per patient day. Payroll expense approached $15 million, about 69 per cent of the total expenditures. Capitalization figures were not available, but it was estimated the total assets of the Indian hospitals were in the neighborhood of $30 million.

The operating expenses of the Clinical Center of the National Institutes of Health were approximately $6.5 million in 1957, or close to $56.00 per patient day. Payroll expenses were around $5.5 million, or roughly 83 per cent of the total. There were no figures available on the amount of capital that was invested in the center.

Patterns of Hospital Ownership and Control

The federal government, through Congressional appropriations, is the primary source of both operating income and capital funds for all Public Health Service institutions.

Educational and Research Activities. None of the sixteen institutions operated by the Division of Hospitals had either a professional or practical nursing school in 1957. However, eight hospitals were approved for residencies and seven for internships by the American Medical Association. In addition, several hospitals offered approved internships for dentists and one had a dietetic internship.

None of the fifty-five Indian hospitals was approved for residencies or internships and none maintained a professional nursing school. Nevertheless, education was playing an important role in these institutions. Practical nursing schools had been established in connection with two hospitals, and dental assistants and technicians were being trained in a number of institutions. Hospital personnel were also working with professional health educators in helping Indian patients and families solve their sanitary, dietary, and other health problems.

As previously indicated, the research arm of the Public Health Service is the National Institutes of Health. All patients must be referred to the Clinical Center by their own physicians and are selected for admission by research investigators to meet the requirements of research projects.

Administration. The head of each of the sixteen hospitals operated by the Division of Hospitals is a commissioned officer in the Public Health Service known as the Medical Officer in Charge (MOC). He is directly responsible to the Chief, Division of Hospitals, for the operation and management of his institution. In general, each of these hospitals is divided internally into clinical and administrative branches respectively headed by a Director of Clinics and an Administrative Officer who are assistants to the MOC.

All of the Indian hospitals are also managed by physicians, most of whom are commissioned officers in the Service. Generally, these Medical Officers in Charge serve in the dual capacity of administrator and medical director. They are responsible to Area Medical Officers in Charge for the operation of their hospitals.

As mentioned earlier, an Assistant Surgeon General is the head of the National Institutes of Health. He reports directly to the Surgeon General of the Public Health Service.

Medical Staff. The medical staff in each of the sixteen institutions operated by the Division of Hospitals is composed of physicians who are commissioned officers in the Service. These staffs are organized by clinical services in a manner similar to that employed in many other hospitals in the United States.

The medical staffs in the larger Indian hospitals are also organized by clinical services; however, such an organization pattern is impractical in many of the smaller institutions which have staffs consisting of just a few physicians.

Saint Elizabeth's Hospital. Saint Elizabeth's Hospital in Washington, D.C., is a separate agency of the Department of Health, Education, and Welfare. It was established in 1855 as the Government Hospital for the Insane and was given its present name in 1916. Originally under the Department of Interior, its functions were transferred to the Federal Security Agency in 1940 and to the newly organized Department of Health, Education, and Welfare in 1953.

Saint Elizabeth's is a long-term, psychiatric hospital providing treatment for several classes of mentally ill persons, including the following: (1) residents of the District of Columbia; (2) beneficiaries of the Veterans Administration; (3) beneficiaries of the Public Health Service; (4) mentally ill persons charged with or convicted of crimes in United States courts; (5) certain American citizens found mentally ill in Canada, the Canal Zone, and the Virgin Islands; (6) certain foreign service personnel; (7) members of the military services admitted to the hospital prior to July 16, 1946.

During 1957 about 1600 patients were admitted to the hospital's 7398 beds. Nearly 7000 patients were in the institution on any given day and the average occupancy rate was roughly 95 per cent. The hospital employed around 2600 persons during the year. Total operating expenses were close to $15 million and payroll expenditures approximated $10.8 million.

Saint Elizabeth's is a member of the American Hospital Association and its respective state and regional association, is accredited by the Joint Commission on Accreditation of Hospitals, is approved by the American Medical Association for internships and residencies. The hospital is also affiliated with a medical school.

Trends. It seems unlikely that the number of persons eligible for admission to the hospitals operated by the Department of Health, Education, and Welfare will increase or decrease markedly in the future. As a result, the number of hospitals and beds should remain relatively constant.

An exception to this general statement might be the institutions controlled by the Division of Indian Health of the Public Health Service. This division is the only section in the Department of Health, Education, and Welfare which is currently engaged in an extensive hospital construction program. The division is building several new Indian hospitals. Some of these will provide new facilities in areas where none existed before, while others are being constructed to replace old, obsolete institutions.

The addition of these new facilities will not significantly increase the present number of hospitals and beds available to the Indian population. However, there is a possibility that through the Public Health Service program of health education, the Indians and Alaskan natives will utilize the hospital facilities more extensively and will create a demand in the future for additional beds and additional hospitals.

State and Local Governmental Hospitals

In 1956 more than 68 per cent of all state hospitals were located east of the Mississippi River. The early settlement and heavier concentration of population in the eastern section of the country are the two most apparent reasons for the unequal distribution of state hospitals east and west of the Mississippi. Every state government operates at least one state hospital and most states place primary emphasis on programs of institutional care and treatment of the mentally ill and tuberculosis patients. New York, Pennsylvania, Massachusetts, Ohio, Illinois, and California maintain the greatest number as might be expected because of their large populations. On the other hand, Nevada, which has fewer people than any other state in the country, operated only one such institution in 1956.

Organizational Structure and Governing Authority. State hospitals are normally controlled by departments, boards, or administrative agencies of the state governments. However, the specific agencies involved vary considerably from state to state; in a state which owns and maintains more than one hospital, operating control may be vested in several different departments or boards.

Most commonly, state hospitals are controlled by departments of health, departments of welfare, boards of charity and correction, or departments of institutions. Special hospital boards or commissions also control a substantial number of state hospitals. Such a commission is generally appointed by the governor with the approval of the state legislature and, beyond submitting a budget for each hospital it controls to the legislature or to an administrative agency or department of the state government, is usually given complete and independent operating authority.

The twenty-odd state university hospitals are normally controlled directly by the medical schools of which they are almost always a part and more indirectly by their respective university's board of regents.

Patterns of Hospital Ownership and Control

Some state hospitals are actually hospital departments of state schools for the blind, deaf, or mentally deficient or of other state institutions such as reformatories and prisons. These hospital departments are controlled by the institutions to which they are attached.

Admission Requirements. Most commonly, patients seeking admission to a state hospital must have been residents of the state for a certain period of time and must be unable to pay for hospitalization on a private basis. However, admission requirements vary from state to state and, depending on the type of medical service rendered, from hospital to hospital.

A basic requirement at many state *university* hospitals is that *all* patients must be referred by their local physicians. Patients at such an institution are often classified, according to their ability to pay for hospital care, as "free," "part-pay," or "full-pay" and additional admission requirements vary, as follows, with the particular classification used.

1. Free Patients. Free patients are normally those who are unable to afford private hospital and medical care. In other words, they are medically indigent. As such, they are almost always the legal responsibility of local units of government, and authorization must usually be obtained from these units before such patients can be admitted to a state university hospital. The cost of caring for these patients is generally shared by the state and the local governmental units.

2. Part-Pay Patients. Part-pay patients have limited financial resources but are not entirely indigent for medical purposes. At a state university hospital, these patients are normally billed for their outpatient clinic and/or hospital expenses but are not charged for the professional services of the medical staff. Prior to admission, such patients and their local physicians are often required to complete a form testifying to the patients' limited financial resources and need for hospitalization.

3. Full-Pay Patients. To supplement their incomes, members of the medical staff at a state university hospital are frequently allowed to admit a limited number of private patients. Such patients are billed for their hospital and/or clinic care and for the professional services of the staff.

A psychiatric patient is usually *committed* to a state mental hospital by a court on the recommendation of a court-appointed board of examiners who have examined and evaluated petitions from the patient's relatives, the testimony of psychiatrists, etc., in a commitment hearing.

History of Growth and Development. Charity Hospital of Louisiana at New Orleans is the oldest of the present state hospitals. It was founded in 1736 when a sailor, Jean Louis, contributed twelve thousand livres ($2500) for this purpose. Originally, it served as both a hospital and a poorhouse, a dual role common in early American hospitals.

Two other state hospitals were also established in the 1700s. Eastern State Hospital in Williamsburg, Virginia, opened in 1773 and Spring Grove State Hospital in Catonsville, Maryland, followed in 1797. The former institution is the oldest hospital in the United States devoted exclusively to the care of the mentally ill. Much of the credit for its founding belongs to Sir Francis Fauquier who, as Governor General of His Majesty's Colony of Virginia, addressed the House of Burgesses in 1766 in these words: "It is expected I should also recommend to your consideration and humanity, a poor, unhappy set of people, who are deprived of their senses and wander about the country terrifying the rest of their fellow creatures. A legal confinement and proper provision ought to be appointed for these miserable objects."

As a result of this eloquent appeal the Burgesses passed a resolution "that a hospital be erected for the reception of persons who are so unhappy as to be deprived of their reason," and, in 1773, the "Public Hospital for Persons of Insane and Disordered Mind" was opened. In 1841 the name was changed to the Eastern Lunatic Asylum and, in 1894, to the Eastern State Hospital.

Soon after their admission to the union the various states were faced with the necessity of providing hospital care for some of their residents, particularly the mentally ill. As a result, many state hospitals began operating during the nineteenth century.

Although a large number of state hospitals — nearly 12 per cent of those in operation in 1956 — opened after World War II, many others closed during the period and the net result was only a slight rise in the total number of such institutions. However, the number of state hospital beds increased by more than 100,000 from 1945 to 1956.

Measures of Significance. In 1956 there were 553 state hospitals in the United States with a combined capacity of 728,151 beds. The average daily census during the year was estimated at nearly 681,000 patients and the average occupancy rate at 93.5 per cent. In the same period there were more than 861,000 admissions to these institutions, or approximately 1.18 admissions per bed. This latter figure is extremely low when compared with other hospital patterns and graphically illustrates the long-term nature of most state hospitals.

Included among these state institutions were 159 general, 271 psychiatric, 93 tuberculosis, and 30 "other" hospitals. Because the majority of state hospitals are usually psychiatric, tuberculosis, or general teaching institutions, they are typically large in capacity. Only 20 per cent of the hospitals had less than 100 beds in 1956 and almost 52 per cent contained 500 beds or more. The average capacity of all state hospitals was over 1316 beds and the average state psychiatric hospital had more than 2427 beds. The six-bed hospital department at the New Jersey State Home for Girls in Trenton, New Jersey, was the smallest state hospital. The 14,742-bed Pilgrim State Hospital in Brentwood, New York, was not only the largest state hospital but was the largest hospital of any kind in the United States and perhaps in the world.

In 1956, nearly 44 per cent of the state hospitals were accredited by the Joint Commission on Accreditation of Hospitals; approximately 46 per cent were members of the American Hospital Association and over 43 per cent belonged to state and/or regional hospital associations.

An estimated 243,180 persons were employed in state hospitals, or only one employee for every 2.8 patients.

Financial Data. The total operating expenses of state hospitals in 1956 were estimated to exceed $1044 million. The cost per patient day was approximately $4.20, which was very low in comparison with other hospital patterns. Payroll expenses were estimated at nearly $668 million, almost 64 per cent of the total operating expenses. In the same year, the total assets of state hospitals were evaluated at more than $2.5 billion, or approximately $3530 per bed.

State hospitals are operated primarily with funds received from the individual state governments. However, some revenue is derived from patients who can afford to pay all or a part of their hospital bill, from foundations and the federal government for research, etc., and from counties and townships for services rendered to their medically indigent in state hospitals. Capital funds are principally obtained from the state governments and from the federal government through Hill-Burton grants.

Educational and Research Activities. As a group, state hospitals are not exceptionally active in either education or research. Less than 29 per cent of the hospitals were approved for residencies by the American Medical Association in 1956 and only 4 per cent offered approved internships. Thirteen per cent maintained affiliations with medical schools, 10 per cent operated approved professional nursing programs, and 4 per cent had approved practical nursing schools.

However, the twenty-odd state university hospitals and the medical schools of which they are usually a part have contributed heavily to the advancement of medical knowledge over the years. These institutions carry on intensive research into all aspects of medical science and medical practice and provide clinical experience and training to large numbers of medical and nursing students at both an undergraduate and graduate level. State university hospitals also maintain schools or courses in nearly all of the paramedical fields.

Administration. The administrator of a state hospital which is controlled by a department, board, or administrative agency of a state government is directly responsible to that department or board for the operation of his institution.

State university hospitals normally operate as part of a medical school, and the administrator of such a hospital generally reports to the medical school dean who, in turn, is responsible to the president of the university and the board of regents.

Hospital departments or infirmaries of prisons, reformatories, and other state institutions are usually under the general direction and control of the head of the institution to which they are attached.

Most state hospitals are administered by physicians who frequently serve in the dual role of superintendent and medical director.

Medical Staff. The medical staff in a state hospital providing general-acute care normally is organized by clinical services under a medical director or, as is often the case in a state university hospital, under the dean of a medical school.

Most state hospitals, however, render only one type of medical service and, consequently, the medical staffs cannot be organized in the above manner. These "special" institutions, particularly the state psychiatric hospitals, often have a large number of beds and house their patients in several different buildings. The medical staff in such a hospital is frequently organized by geographical area with each physician on the staff being assigned to care for the patients in a certain building or buildings.

Usually, the medical staff in a state hospital is composed of physicians who are full-time salaried employees of the hospital. They are often appointed to their positions by a state civil service commission and are subject to the same rules and regulations as other state governmental employees. Private practitioners are frequently used as consultants but are generally not eligible for staff membership in a state hospital on any other basis.

Full-time physicians at a state university hospital normally hold academic appointments in the university's medical school. To supplement their salaries, these physicians, as previously mentioned, are often allowed to admit a limited number of private patients to the hospital.

Trends. State governments will always find it necessary to provide hospital facilities for some of their residents, particularly the mentally ill whose care has traditionally been a responsibility of the various states. The length of stay (long-term care) for this type of illness and for other chronic diseases means that the average person will not be able to finance such an illness. Consequently, as the population of the United States continues to grow, the number of hospitals and beds maintained by state governments should gradually increase — though the size of the individual units will be smaller in order to develop a superior pattern for care — and more patients will thus be enabled to receive modern medical care nearer to their homes.

Hospital districts are political subdivisions created for the purpose of establishing and maintaining a hospital. They have the advantage of meeting the need for suburban and rural hospital facilities on a local level without external government controls and, at the same time, they contain a taxable population which is large enough to insure adequate financing for the construction and maintenance of a hospital.

Geographically, one county may contain several hospital districts or the reverse may be true where one hospital district has within its boundaries all or part of two or more counties.

The procedure for establishing a hospital district varies with the individual states. In California, which contained nearly 25 per cent of all the district hospitals in the United States in 1956, the creation of a hospital district — an action taken under general state enabling acts — follows three steps: (1) petition by the residents; (2) examination of the petition by a local board of county supervisors; (3) approval at an election in the proposed district.

Organizational Structure and Governing Authority. The affairs of a hospital district are usually governed by a board of directors elected by the residents of the district for terms of from two to four years. The board is also responsible for operating the district hospital; in this capacity its functions are almost identical with those of a board of trustees in a voluntary, nonprofit, nongovernmental hospital.

History of Growth and Development. Special school, airport, conservation, sanitary, water, and utility districts are very common in the United States and have been used extensively for many years. However, only in recent years have special hospital districts been employed to any great degree.

Several of the present district hospitals were established as far back as the turn of the century. However, it is not known whether they were originally controlled and maintained by hospital districts. It is possible they opened under a different ownership pattern and, at a later date, were taken over by hospital districts.

Less than 20 per cent of the district hospitals in operation in 1956 were established prior to 1940 and nearly 72 per cent opened after World War II.

Measures of Significance. In 1956 there were ninety-one district hospitals in the United States, with a combined capacity of 7724 beds.

During the year they admitted an estimated 240,000 patients, or approximately 31 admissions per bed. The average daily census was nearly 5100 patients and the average occupancy rate was about 66 per cent.

Six of the district hospitals provided long-term care for tuberculosis patients and one was a long-term chronic disease and convalescent institution. All of the remaining district hospitals provided short-term, general-acute care.

District hospitals are generally quite small. In 1956 the average capacity was approximately 85 beds. Over 67 per cent of the hospitals had less than 100 beds and only two hospitals contained 300 beds or more. The largest district hospital was the 783-bed institution operated by the Dallas County Hospital District in Dallas, Texas.

Nearly 36 per cent of the hospitals were accredited by the Joint Commission on Accreditation of Hospitals. Approximately 85 per cent were members of the American Hospital Association and more than 92 per cent belonged to state and/or regional associations.

Over 10,300 persons were employed in district hospitals in 1956, or slightly more than two employees per patient.

District hospitals were located in only fifteen of the forty-eight states during that year and nearly 73 per cent were concentrated in five states: California, Washington, Illinois, Kansas, and Florida. Approximately 62 per cent of the hospitals were west of the Mississippi River and the American Hospital Association's Pacific region alone contained close to 46 per cent of the total number in the United States.

Financial Data. Total assets of the district hospitals were estimated to exceed $85 million, or slightly more than $11,000 per bed. Capital funds are primarily obtained from the federal and state governments and from the sale of bonds issued upon the approval of the voters of the district.

In 1956 the operating expenses of district hospitals were estimated to exceed $45 million, or nearly $25.00 per patient day. Estimated payroll expenditures were more than $28 million and the payroll component of total expenses was approximately 62 per cent. District hospitals, unlike many of the institutions operated by other governmental units, were principally established to serve the paying patient; they normally provide only a small amount of free service to the medically indigent. As a result, patient revenue is the primary source of operating income.

Hospital districts have the authority to levy taxes. Some districts have never found it necessary to levy a tax, while others use tax revenue to balance hospital operating income and expense. Tax funds are also used occasionally to pay the interest on any outstanding bonds of the hospital district and/or to accumulate a sinking fund for the payment of the principal when the bonds have matured.

Educational Activities. District hospitals are not very active in the area of education. Undoubtedly, this is principally due to the fact that most of the hospitals are quite small and are unable to support educational programs to any great degree. Only four hospitals had been approved for residency training by the American Medical Association in 1956. Two hospitals were approved for internships and two were affiliated with medical schools. One hospital operated an approved professional nursing school.

Administration. The operation of a district hospital is normally in the hands of a nonmedical administrator. He coordinates his functions with the medical director and is responsible to the board of directors of the hospital district.

Medical Staff. Medical staff membership in district hospitals is usually open to all qualified doctors of medicine and, in some of the hospitals, is also open to licensed doctors of osteopathy. In the larger hospitals the staff is generally organized by clinical services under a medical director.

Trends. District hospitals are growing at a proportionately faster rate than any other hospital pattern. In the two-year period from 1954 to 1956, the number of district hospitals in the United States increased from 68 to 91 and the bed capacity almost doubled.

Although district hospitals were located in only fifteen states in 1956, statutes permitting the establishment of hospital districts had been enacted by several other state legislatures. Consequently, it seems reasonable to expect that district hospitals will continue to grow at a rapid pace in the future. By overcoming the limits of local government boundaries, district ownership becomes an appealing pattern.

COUNTY HOSPITALS

County hospitals constitute one of the more important patterns of hospital ownership and control. Approximately one out of every ten hospitals in the United States in 1956 was owned and maintained by a county government. In addition, more than 32 per cent of the various governmental hospitals were county institutions.

Organizational Structure and Governing Authority. County hospitals are controlled in a number of different ways. A few hospitals are the direct responsibility of a county board of supervisors or commissioners. Other county hospitals are supervised by a county welfare board or department. A separate hospital board composed of representative citizens of the county is perhaps the most common form of control. The members of such a board may be appointed by the county board of supervisors or may be elected to their positions. In either case, they generally have complete authority to operate the hospital, although the institution's annual budget must usually be approved by the county board of supervisors. The following examples illustrate two variations in the organization and control of county hospitals.

Itasca Memorial Hospital, Grand Rapids, Minnesota. Itasca County is governed by a board of county commissioners composed of five members elected from the various districts within the county. Each of the five commissioners appoints one person from his district to serve on the county welfare board, which is responsible for the care of the poor, the tubercular, and the medically indigent. The welfare board also is responsible for the "complete and exclusive control, care, management, maintenance, and operation" of the county hospital and, in this regard, functions in the same way as the board of trustees in a nonprofit, nongovernmental hospital.

Los Angeles County General Hospital, Los Angeles, California. Los Angeles County is one of the most populous counties in the United States. It has an elaborate and complex organizational structure and employs more than 32,000 persons to perform the variety of public services it renders.

The county is divided into five districts. Each district elects one representative to serve on the Board of Supervisors, which is the governing body of the county. The term of office is four years. The Chief Administrative Officer, appointed by the board for an indefinite term, is directly responsible to the Board of Supervisors for the management of the county.

Los Angeles County General Hospital and the other hospitals operated by the county are under the general direction and control of the Superintendent of Charities as head of the Department of Charities. He makes the final appointment of the various hospital directors and is responsible to the Chief Administrative Officer for the operation of his department.

Admission Requirements. County hospitals are similar to the city and city-county hospital patterns in their admission requirements. Many county hospitals, particularly those located in metropolitan areas, were primarily established to serve the medically indigent, who must meet certain financial and residence requirements before they are eligible for admission. In these institutions, "private" patients are usually admitted only in case of emergency or for the treatment of specific conditions.

The remaining county hospitals are principally concerned with the care and treatment of paying patients. These institutions generally do not have any special requirements which must be met before a patient can be admitted.

History of Growth and Development. The oldest county hospital in the United States is the Wayne County Hospital and Infirmary in Eloise, Michigan, opened in 1833. A large number of other county hospitals — nearly 9 per cent of those in operation in 1956 — were also established prior to 1900, particularly in the states of California and Wisconsin.

The number of county hospitals increased at a gradual but steady pace from 1900 to 1945. With the end of World War II, their rate of growth accelerated and roughly 42 per cent of the county hospitals in operation in 1956 opened during this period. Undoubtedly, much of this latter growth was due to the federal grants for hospital construction received under the terms of the Hill-Burton Act of 1946. The southern states, in particular, have benefited from this act; a high proportion of the newly established county hospitals are located in the southern section of the country. In the state of Texas alone, fifty-three such institutions were founded in the interval from 1946 to 1956.

Measures of Significance. In 1956 there were 722 county hospitals in the United States with a combined capacity of 114,760 beds. There were an estimated 1.6 million admissions to these hospitals during the year, or approximately 14 admissions per bed. The average daily census was estimated at nearly 90,000 patients; the average occupancy rate was around 78 per cent.

Over 73 per cent of the county hospitals were general-acute institutions and more than 18 per cent were primarily concerned with the treatment of tuberculosis. Psychiatric hospitals accounted for less than 4 per cent of the total and the remaining 4.5 per cent provided chronic, convalescent, and other types of hospital care.

County hospitals had an average capacity of approximately 159 beds in 1956. Nearly 65 per cent of the hospitals had less than 100 beds and only a little over 5 per cent contained 500 beds or more. The oldest county hospital — Wayne County General Hospital and Infirmary in Eloise, Michigan — was also the largest, with 6931 beds. The smallest was the eight-bed Edwards County Memorial Hospital in Rocksprings, Texas.

In 1956, 257 county hospitals, or slightly less than 36 per cent of the total, were accredited by the Joint Commission on Accreditation of Hospitals. Over 68 per cent were members of the American Hospital Association and approximately 74 per cent were participating in state and/or regional hospital associations.

An estimated 119,000 persons were employed in county hospitals during the year, or about 1.3 employees per patient.

County hospitals are scattered throughout the United States and can be found in each of the nine geographic regions established by the American Hospital Association. More than 59 per cent of the hospitals in 1956 were east of the Mississippi River and the East North Central region (Ohio, Indiana, Illinois, Michigan, and Wisconsin) was particularly well endowed with institutions of this kind. Only eleven county hospitals, or less than 2 per cent of the total, were contained in the New England region. This is probably explained by the fact that, in this part of the country, the township — not the county — is and always has been the principal form of local government. Among the individual states, Texas and California had 76 and 56 county hospitals respectively while eight states (Maine, Vermont, Rhode Island, Connecticut, Delaware, Virginia, North Dakota, and Louisiana) contained no institutions of this type.

Financial Data. County hospitals expended an estimated $512 million during 1956, or approximately $15.70 per patient day. Payroll expenditures in the same year exceeded $353 million and the payroll component of total expenses was over 69 per cent. Total assets were estimated at more than $975 million, or about $8500 per bed.

The county government is the principal source of operating income in those hospitals which are primarily devoted to the care of the medically indigent. However, most county hospitals were established to serve a paying clientele. In these institutions, almost all operating income is derived from patients and very little is received from the county. Capital funds for construction and expansion are generally obtained from the various county governments and from federal grants.

Educational Activities. Among the county hospitals in the United States are such famous teaching institutions as Cook County Hospital in Chicago, Illinois, and Los Angeles County General Hospital in Los Angeles, California. However, as a group, county hospitals are not very active in the area of education. Less than 9 per cent were approved for residency training by the American Medical Association in 1956, and only 5 per cent were approved for internships. Eighteen, or just over 2 per cent of the hospitals, were affiliated with medical schools. Thirty-two county hospitals had approved professional nursing schools and approved practical nursing programs were in operation in thirty-three hospitals.

Administration. Most of the smaller county hospitals are managed by a nonmedical administrator who is directly responsible to the commission, board of control, or other body governing the hospital. The top administrative position in some of the larger hospitals is held by a member of the medical profession who usually assumes the duties of both superintendent and medical director.

Medical Staff. County hospitals are similar to the city-county hospital pattern in the composition and organization of their medical staffs. Those hospitals which are primarily concerned with the care of the

77

medically indigent usually have active medical education programs. In such an institution the medical staff generally includes several physicians who serve at the hospital on a full-time basis and whose principal duties are to instruct and supervise the medical clerks, interns, and residents. The remainder of the staff normally consists of private practitioners. Though they usually must admit their own patients to other hospitals in the area, these physicians voluntarily serve the county hospital in caring for the medically indigent and in assisting with the instruction and supervision of the residents, interns, and medical students.

Most of the other county hospitals were established to serve paying patients. The medical staffs in these institutions function in the same way as the staffs in most nonprofit, nongovernmental hospitals.

Trends. As stated previously, there has been a remarkable increase in the number of county hospitals since the end of World War II. This is illustrated by the fact that approximately 42 per cent of the county hospitals in operation in 1956 were established after 1945. However, it appears that their rate of growth is beginning to level off. In the future, county hospitals will increase in number but at a much slower pace than in recent years. As the suburban populations of large cities increase faster than the city populations, many services will be financed on a county basis rather than on a city basis. Hence, some city hospitals will eventually become county hospitals.

CITY-COUNTY HOSPITALS

City-county hospitals are local governmental institutions controlled jointly by municipal and county governments. They are established primarily as a means of sharing the financial burden of hospital construction and operation including, particularly in metropolitan areas, the care of the medically indigent.

Organizational Structure and Governing Authority. There is considerable variance among city-county hospitals in the manner in which they are organized and controlled. Usually, such an institution is governed by a hospital board of control. One half of the board members are normally appointed by the mayor and/or the city council and one half by the county board of commissioners and/or the county judge. The hospital board almost always has complete authority to operate the hospital, although the institution's annual budget must generally be approved by both city and county representatives. The following example briefly illustrates one of the many different organizational patterns occurring in city-county hospitals.

Ancker Hospital, St. Paul, Minnesota. Ancker Hospital is a city-county institution governed by the Ramsey County Welfare Board.

The mayor of St. Paul appoints all five board members; however, the appointment of two members is subject to the approval of the city council and three appointees must be approved by the county commissioners. Members of the board serve three-year terms and are prohibited from holding political office during their tenure.

Admission Requirements. A significant number of city-county hospitals are located in metropolitan areas and were established primarily as a means of lessening the burden to the private hospitals of the cost of caring for the medically indigent and to provide this care at a level which would result in less cost to the taxpayer. In these hospitals the medically indigent must usually meet both a financial and a residence requirement. In other words, they must be unable to pay for "private" hospital care and must have resided in the city or county for a certain period of time. "Private" patients are generally admitted to these hospitals only in case of emergency or for the treatment of specific ailments (contagious diseases, psychiatric disorders, and others) which other hospitals in the area are not prepared to handle.

Most of the other city-county hospitals provide very little service to the medically indigent. They derive most of their income from paying patients and have no specific requirements, other than the need for hospitalization, which must be met before patients can be admitted.

History of Growth and Development. Louisville General Hospital in Louisville, Kentucky, was established in 1817 and is the oldest of the present city-county hospitals. Three others opened prior to the Civil War and twelve city-county hospitals were in operation at the turn of the century. From 1900 to 1940, city-county hospitals increased in both size and number at a gradual but steady rate. Since 1940 they have grown at an accelerated pace; thirty-two of the city-county hospitals in operation in 1956 were established during this period.

Measures of Significance. In 1956 there were eighty-five city-county hospitals in the United States. They had a combined capacity of 13,944 beds and, during the year, admitted an estimated 353,480 patients, or over 25 admissions per bed. The average daily census in the same period was estimated at 10,119 patients and the average occupancy rate was nearly 73 per cent.

The eighty-five hospitals included nine long-term and seventy-six short-term institutions. Seventy-five hospitals provided general-acute care; eight were primarily concerned with the treatment of tuberculosis; one was a children's hospital; and one was a chronic disease and convalescent institution.

In 1956, city-county hospitals had an average capacity of over 164 beds. Forty-eight hospitals, or nearly 57 per cent of the total, had less than 100 beds and only seven had 500 beds or more. They ranged in size from 20 to 1132 beds, the largest being the San Francisco Hospital in San Francisco, California.

In the same year, forty-four hospitals held accreditation by the Joint Commission on Accreditation of Hospitals, sixty-eight were members of the American Hospital Association, and seventy-nine — or almost 93 per cent of the total — belonged to state and/or regional hospital associations.

An estimated 16,872 persons were employed in city-county hospitals in 1956, or approximately 1.67 employees per patient.

With the exception of the New England region, all nine geographic areas established by the American Hospital Association contained at least one city-county hospital in 1956. Nearly 66 per cent of the hospitals were located east of the Mississippi River, particularly in the southeast section of the United States. Twenty-five states had no city-county hospitals while Georgia and Texas each had fourteen.

Financial Data. Total expenditures of city-county hospitals in 1956 were estimated to exceed $66.5 million or just over $18.00 per patient day. Estimated payroll expenses were around $41.5 million and the payroll component of total expenses was over 62 per cent. In the same year, total assets were estimated at more than $118 million, or roughly $8500 per bed.

In most of the city-county hospitals, paying patients are the primary source of operating income. However, in those hospitals which were established principally to serve the medically indigent, the city and county governments provide most of the operating income and only a small percentage is derived from paying patients. Capital funds for construction and expansion are obtained from the two units of government and from federal grants.

Educational Activities. The American Medical Association approved fifteen city-county hospitals for residency training and fourteen for internships in 1956. In addition, nine hospitals were affiliated with medical schools. Seventeen, or 20 per cent of the hospitals, had approved professional nursing schools and eight hospitals operated approved practical nursing programs.

Administration. A nonmedical administrator holds the top executive position in most city-county hospitals. He coordinates his functions with the medical director or chief of staff and is responsible to the board of control, board of commissioners, or other body governing the hospital.

Some of the larger city-county hospitals are administered by physicians who usually serve in the dual capacity of administrator and medical director.

Medical Staff. Many of the larger city-county hospitals which are primarily devoted to the care of the medically indigent are also extremely active in the area of medical education. The medical staff generally includes a number of physicians who are employed at the hospital on a full-time basis. They are not only concerned with the care and treatment of patients but also instruct and supervise the medical clerks, interns, and residents in training at the hospital. The balance of the medical staff is normally composed of physicians who are engaged in private practice in the area. Although their private patients are usually not eligible for admission to the hospital, these practitioners find satisfaction in caring for the medically indigent and in supervising and instructing the residents, interns, and medical students. Also, their affiliation with a teaching institution enables these physicians to advance their own professional knowledge.

Most of the other city-county hospitals were principally established to serve the paying patient, and the medical staff in such an institution functions in the same way as the staff in a nonprofit, nongovernmental hospital.

Trends. There has been a considerable increase in the number of city-county hospitals in recent years. It seems reasonable to assume this growth will continue because of the advantages — local control and a wide taxation base — inherent in this type of hospital. However, district hospitals offer the same advantages and their remarkable increase in the past few years may be an indication that the trend is away from city-county hospitals. In the future, city and county governments which desire to establish a hospital may prefer to create a district hospital rather than a city-county institution.

CITY HOSPITALS

Hospitals owned and maintained by municipal governments accounted for more than 5 per cent of all hospitals in the United States in 1956 and for nearly 6 per cent of all hospital admissions. In addition, approximately one of every six governmental hospitals in this country was a city institution.

Organizational Structure and Governing Authority. City hospitals vary a great deal in their organizational structure and in the manner in which they are controlled and maintained. Some are operated as a division of a department or board of the city government, usually that department or board which is responsible for health and/or welfare activities. In cities maintaining more than one municipal hospital, operating control may be vested in a separate "Department of Hospitals." The city manager or mayor controls the city hospital in some communities. In other cities, the municipal hospital is the responsibility of the city council or a committee of the council.

A separate hospital board or commission, composed of representative

81

citizens of the community, is perhaps the most common form of controlling city hospitals. Board members are generally appointed rather than elected to their positions, and the appointments are usually made by the mayor and/or the city council. Normally, such a board is relatively free of political interference and has complete authority over the operation of the city hospital. However, the institution's annual budget may be subject to the review and approval of the city council. The following example illustrates one of the many variations in the organization and control of city hospitals.

Minneapolis General Hospital, Minneapolis, Minnesota. The Minneapolis General Hospital is a separate department of the Board of Public Welfare, which is also responsible for the health and relief departments and the city workhouse. The board consists of seven members — the mayor, two aldermen selected by the city council, and four persons representing industry, labor, the medical profession, and the general public — who are appointed by the mayor with the approval of the city council. The aldermen serve two-year terms on the board. The mayor's appointees serve four-year terms which are staggered so that one person is selected each year.

The hospital is administered by a nonmedical superintendent who reports directly to the board. The hospital's annual budget is reviewed by the finance committee of the welfare board and is then submitted to the ways and means committee of the city council for final approval.

Admission Requirements. Most city hospitals serve a paying clientele, and patients seeking admission to these institutions usually do not have to meet any specific requirements.

The situation is different, however, in the municipal hospitals which were established to provide care to the medically indigent. To be eligible for admission to these institutions on a free basis, patients generally must be unable to pay for "private" hospital and medical care and also must have resided in the city for a certain period of time. These hospitals normally accept "private" or paying patients only in case of emergency or for the treatment of certain conditions which other hospitals in the area are not prepared to handle.

History of Growth and Development. The Philadelphia General Hospital, Blockley Division, in Philadelphia, Pennsylvania, is not only the oldest *city* hospital but, in terms of its founding date, is also the oldest of *all* the hospitals currently in operation in the United States. It was established in 1732 and was originally maintained as a public almshouse or poorhouse for the aged, the infirm, and the insane. For many years the only treatment facility in the institution was a small infirmary where inmates requiring medical attention were seen by local physicians. Eventually, in 1781, "Old Blockley," as it was popularly known, expanded its program to include hospital care.

Two other city hospitals also opened during the eighteenth century. The Bellevue Hospital Center, one of the many municipal hospitals operated by New York City, had its origin in 1736 as The New York Public Workhouse. The Baltimore City Hospital was established in Baltimore, Maryland, in 1776.

Of the city hospitals in operation in 1956, nearly 13 per cent were opened by 1900. Most of these early hospitals are located in New York and the New England states in which the city or town has been the principal form of local government since colonial times.

City hospitals slowly but steadily increased in number from 1900 to 1945. Following World War II, a large number of city hospitals opened but an equal number closed in the same period and many others reduced their bed capacity. As a result, there were 15,000 *fewer* beds in city hospitals in 1956 than there were in 1944.

Measures of Significance. In 1956 the 365 city hospitals in the United States had a combined capacity of 65,940 beds. There were an estimated 1,252,860 admissions to these institutions during the year, or approximately 19 admissions per bed. The average daily census was estimated to exceed 51,400 patients; the average occupancy rate was approximately 78 per cent.

The hospitals included 323 general-acute, two psychiatric, and twelve tuberculosis institutions. The remaining twenty-eight hospitals provided specialized care for chronic illnesses, contagious diseases, and a variety of other medical conditions.

Average capacity of the city hospitals was around 181 beds. They ranged in size from two eight-bed institutions — the Browns Valley Community Hospital in Browns Valley, Minnesota, and the Alcohol Treatment Center in Madison, Wisconsin — to the 3221-bed Kings County Hospital Center in Brooklyn, which was one of nearly thirty hospitals and related facilities operated and maintained by New York City. Over 68 per cent of the city hospitals had fewer than 100 beds. Only thirty-three hospitals — less than one tenth of the total number — contained 500 beds or more.

About 45 per cent of the city hospitals were accredited by the Joint Commission on Accreditation of Hospitals. More than 77 per cent were members of the American Hospital Association and close to 84 per cent belonged to state and/or regional associations.

An estimated 85,000 persons were employed in the 365 city hospitals, or approximately 1.65 employees per patient.

City hospitals are fairly well scattered throughout the entire United States. They are contained in every American Hospital Association geographic region and are almost evenly divided east and west of the Mississippi River. They are most heavily concentrated in the midwestern part of the country in the East North Central and West North Central regions which, in 1956, had eighty and ninety city hospitals respectively. Their lightest concentration was in the Pacific region — Washington, Oregon, and California — which contained only six municipal hospitals or less than 2 per cent of the total number. Five states had no city hospitals while Minnesota and New York each had thirty-nine such institutions. In Minnesota, city hospitals accounted for nearly one fifth of all the hospitals in the state.

Financial Data. It was estimated that over $362 million were expended by city hospitals in 1956, or around $19.30 per patient day. Payroll expenses exceeded $242 million and the payroll component of total expenses was just under 67 per cent.

Total assets in the same year were estimated at $619 million, or approximately $9400 per bed.

Patient revenue is the primary source of operating income in those city hospitals having mainly a paying clientele. In the hospitals which were principally established to serve the medically indigent, the city government provides most of the operating income and only a small proportion is derived from paying patients.

Educational Activities. The American Medical Association approved nearly 18 per cent of the city hospitals for residency training in 1956, and about 13 per cent were approved for internships. Approximately 9 per cent were affiliated with medical schools, 12 per cent operated approved professional nursing programs, and more than 3 per cent had approved practical nursing schools.

Administration. Most city hospitals are managed by a nonmedical administrator who reports directly to the board, commission, or department governing the institution. Some of the larger institutions which have active medical education programs are administered by a physician who generally serves in the dual capacity of superintendent and medical director.

Medical Staff. Composition of the medical staff in a city hospital largely depends, as is also true of the county and city-county hospital patterns, on whether the hospital serves paying patients also or is a teaching institution devoted solely to the care of the medically indigent.

In a city hospital with a large number of indigent patients and an active medical education program the medical staff normally includes several physicians who are employed at the hospital on a full-time basis. They provide some direct patient care but are primarily concerned with the instruction and supervision of the interns, residents, and medical students. The balance of the staff in such an institution is made up of private practitioners who — though they usually receive no compensation for their services and must generally admit their own private patients to other hospitals — care for the medically indigent and assist with the supervision and education of the interns and residents.

In a city hospital which serves both indigent and paying clientele, the medical staff is composed of physicians with private practices who use the hospital, as do staff members of most voluntary hospitals, as a place for treating and caring for their patients.

In both types of city hospitals, the medical staffs are organized by clinical services if size permits.

Trends. As indicated previously, a large number of city hospitals opened after World War II. However, an equal number closed during that period and many others reduced their bed capacity. From 1954 to 1956 both the number of beds and the number of city hospitals decreased significantly. A further decrease seems indicated for the next several years. At the end of that time, however, the decline should begin to level off, and from then on, the number of hospitals and beds operated by city governments should remain relatively constant. For many communities this pattern remains the easiest method of securing capital funds and operating funds.

PART II · NONGOVERNMENTAL PATTERNS

Nothing is little to him that feels it with great sensibility.

SAMUEL JOHNSON

Individualities may form communities, but it is institutions alone that can create a nation.

BENJAMIN DISRAELI

Nongovernmental Hospitals and Their Significance

Mᴏʀᴇ than two thirds of the hospitals in the United States are nongovernmental institutions (see Table 10). They are owned and operated by nonprofit associations and corporations or by proprietary profit-making enterprises rather than by agencies or departments of governmental units. Although nongovernmental hospitals contain less than one third of the nation's total hospital beds, they annually admit nearly three fourths of all hospital patients. In addition, they account for roughly one half of all hospital assets, expenses, and personnel.

NONPROFIT HOSPITALS

The nongovernmental, nonprofit hospitals in the United States form what is commonly referred to as our "voluntary hospital system." These institutions may be divided into two major groups, "church" hospitals and "other nonprofit" hospitals, each of which will be summarized briefly in the following pages.

Approximately one half of the nation's hospitals are nonprofit institutions (see Table 11). Although they contain just over one fourth of the total hospital beds, they admit more than two thirds of all hospital patients. Nonprofit hospitals also account for nearly one half of all hospital assets, expenses, and personnel. As illustrated in the preceding table, their effect on the nongovernmental hospital picture is even more noticeable. They represent almost three fourths of all nongovernmental hospitals and account for roughly 90 per cent of all nongovernmental hospital beds, admissions, assets, expenses, and personnel.

CHURCH HOSPITALS

Church hospitals are institutions owned and/or operated by or related to religious organizations. They include both Roman Catholic and Protestant hospitals. However, they exclude Jewish hospitals which,

89

Patterns of Hospital Ownership and Control

Table 10. Comparison of Nongovernmental Hospitals with All
Continental United States Hospitals in 1956

	Nongov. Total	% of U.S. Total
Number of hospitals	4,718	67.7
Number of beds	493,050	30.7
Average daily census	363,527	26.9
Annual admissions	16,371,087	74.1
Number of paid personnel	725,869	52.8
Assets	$6,464,614,000	49.6
Annual expenses	$3,122,753,000	51.9
Annual payroll expenses...........	$1,888,660,000	47.8

Table 11. Comparison of Nonprofit Hospitals with Nongovernmental
Hospitals and All Continental United States Hospitals in 1956

	Nonprofit Total	% of Nongov. Total	% of U.S. Total
Number of hospitals	3,510	74.4	50.4
Number of beds	442,605	89.8	27.5
Average daily census *	330,141	90.8	24.4
Annual admissions *	14,804,385	90.4	67.0
Number of paid personnel *...	673,904	92.8	49.0
Assets *	$6,247,645,000	96.6	47.9
Annual expenses *	$2,892,855,000	92.6	48.1
Annual payroll expenses *....	$1,765,599,000	93.5	44.7

* Estimated.

though sponsored by members of the Jewish faith, are not affiliated in their ownership or control with Jewish religious bodies.

Vitally important throughout the course of hospital history, church hospitals are no less significant today. In the United States, for example, they currently account for more than one out of every six hospitals and admit over one fourth of all hospital patients (see Table 12).

Roman Catholic hospitals, discussed in the following chapter, are especially significant. They are not only prominent in the church hospital scene but have a tremendous impact on the total hospital industry.

More than 5 per cent of the nation's hospitals are owned and/or operated by Protestant denominations or agencies or are related to such groups. Protestant hospitals are fairly well scattered and all but seven states (Connecticut, Delaware, Maine, Nevada, New Hampshire, Rhode Island, and Vermont) had at least one such institution in 1956. However, they are naturally most heavily concentrated in areas with large Protestant populations, particularly the West North Central region, which alone contains almost one third of all the Protestant hospitals in the country.

Each of the following Protestant denominations is known to own and/or operate or to be affiliated in some manner with one or more hospitals: American Baptist; Southern Baptist; Southwest Baptist; Christian Reformed; Church of Jesus Christ of Latter-Day Saints; Episcopal; Evangelical and Reformed; Evangelical United Brethren; Evangelical Mission Covenant; American Lutheran; Augustana Lutheran; Evangelical Lutheran; Lutheran Free Church; Lutheran Church, Missouri Synod; Methodist; Mennonite; Presbyterian; United Presbyterian; Salvation Army; Seventh-Day Adventist.

A lack of complete and accurate information prevented an individual discussion of the hospitals of each of the above denominations. However, separate discussions in the chapter on nonprofit, church-affiliated hospitals are devoted to the Lutheran, Methodist, Presbyterian, Baptist, and Latter-Day Saints institutions, which are fairly representative of most Protestant patterns of hospital ownership and control.

OTHER NONPROFIT HOSPITALS

Other nonprofit hospitals account for approximately one third of all hospitals in the United States and about one sixth of the total hospital

Table 12. Comparison of Church-Affiliated Hospitals with Nonprofit, Nongovernmental, and All Continental United States Hospitals in 1956

	Church-Affiliated Total	% of Nonprofit Total	% of Nongov. Total	% of U.S. Total
Number of hospitals	1,206	34.4	25.6	17.3
Number of beds	176,972	40.0	35.9	11.0
Average daily census*	132,623	40.2	36.5	9.8
Annual admissions*	6,275,993	42.4	38.3	28.4

* Estimated.

Table 13. Comparison of "Other Nonprofit" Hospitals with Nonprofit, Nongovernmental, and All Continental United States Hospitals in 1956

	"Other Nonprofit" Total	% of Nonprofit Total	% of Nongov. Total	% of U.S. Total
Number of hospitals	2,304	65.6	48.8	33.1
Number of beds	265,633	60.0	53.9	16.5
Average daily census*	197,968	60.0	54.5	14.6
Annual admissions*	8,530,644	57.6	52.1	38.6

* Estimated.

beds (see Table 13). In addition, they admit nearly four out of every ten hospital patients.

The "other nonprofit" category includes hospitals owned and/or operated by such organizations as philanthropic foundations, labor unions, cooperative and other health insurance plans, fraternal societies, industrial enterprises, and employee beneficial associations. Jewish hospitals, the product of Jewish communities rather than of Jewish religious bodies, are also included in this category. However, the vast majority of the "other nonprofit" hospitals are sponsored, not by members of a specific religious faith or by already existing groups similar to those above which were originally organized for other purposes, but by voluntary, nonprofit hospital associations or corporations composed of public-spirited citizens who are interested in providing hospital care for their community and who are organized solely for that purpose. In total, these latter groups own and/or operate more than 2000 so-called community hospitals with a combined capacity of roughly 230,000 beds.

The concluding chapter is devoted to individual discussions of community, Jewish, industrial, cooperative, United Mine Workers, Kaiser Foundation, and Shriners hospitals which are among the more important and better known "other nonprofit" patterns of hospital ownership and control.

PROPRIETARY HOSPITALS

Proprietary hospitals are privately owned and managed institutions which are operated on a "profit," as opposed to a "nonprofit" basis. In other words, they are private business ventures and all or a portion of any operating surplus may revert to their owners.

Proprietary hospitals are often condemned for having, as their critics claim, mercenary and ulterior motives in a field that is normally benevolent in nature. However, only a small proportion of these institutions are deserving of such criticism. Proprietary hospitals are, in reality, an extremely important source of hospital care in this country and are the *only* source of such care in many rural areas. The significance of proprietary hospitals is best illustrated by the fact that, in 1956, they accounted for approximately 17 per cent of all hospitals in the United States and nearly 26 per cent of all the nongovernmental hospitals.

Organizational Structure and Governing Authority. Most proprietary hospitals are owned and controlled by one or more physicians who both administer and staff their respective institutions.

In 1956, approximately 39 per cent of the proprietary hospitals were owned by individuals, 23 per cent by partnerships, and 37 per cent by corporations. Some of the corporate hospitals have a large number of stockholders and, in such a case, a board of ten to twelve directors is often appointed or elected by the stockholders, to manage the affairs of the corporation.

History of Growth and Development. Sufficient data are not available to closely trace the history of proprietary hospitals. It is estimated that there were less than 100 such institutions in the United States at the turn of the century and that by 1928 nearly 2500 proprietary hospitals were in existence. From then on, the number of proprietary hospitals began to decline.

Several factors influenced the phenomenal growth of these proprietary institutions in the first thirty years of the twentieth century. First of all, voluntary organizations and state and local governments in some sections of the country, particularly the south and southwest, neglected their responsibilities in providing adequate hospital facilities, and physicians in these areas were forced to establish hospitals of their own. Secondly, a number of proprietary hospitals were founded by physicians who desired to control all aspects of their medical practice and who felt unnecessarily hampered and regulated in other types of hospitals. Finally, many proprietary hospitals were opened for no other reason than the expectation of earning a financial profit.

Measures of Significance. There were 1208 proprietary hospitals in the United States in 1956. During the year, nearly 1,589,000 patients were admitted to the 50,447 beds contained in these hospitals, or nearly 32 patients per bed. The average daily census in the same period was 33,368 patients; the average occupancy rate was roughly 66 per cent.

Almost 78 per cent of these proprietary hospitals were general-acute institutions. Twelve per cent were psychiatric hospitals, 1 per cent specialized in the treatment of tuberculosis, and the remaining 9 per cent were "other special" hospitals.

Proprietary hospitals are typically very small. In 1956 they had an average capacity of under 42 beds, and 446 of the hospitals — or nearly 37 per cent — had less than 25 beds. The largest hospital had 520 beds and was the only proprietary hospital containing 300 beds or more. Generally, the smallest proprietary hospitals are those owned by individuals and partnerships. The corporate institutions are somewhat larger.

An estimated 14 per cent of the proprietary hospitals were accredited by the Joint Commission on Accreditation of Hospitals. Data were not available on the number of proprietary institutions that belonged to the American Hospital Association or to state and/or regional associations; however, it is believed a substantial proportion of proprietary hospitals were members of these groups.

Nearly 52,000 persons were employed in proprietary hospitals in 1956, or approximately 1.6 employees per patient.

In the same year, proprietary hospitals were located in every geographic region of the American Hospital Association and in every state in the union except Delaware, New Hampshire, and North Dakota. However, they were most heavily concentrated in the South Atlantic, East South Central, and West South Central regions, which together contained almost 65 per cent of the proprietary hospitals in the United States. Proprietary institutions accounted for nearly one third of all the hospitals in Alabama, Arkansas, Tennessee, and West Virginia, and close to one half of all the hospitals in Texas and Louisiana. Texas alone had more than 250 proprietary hospitals, or about 21 per cent of all such hospitals in the nation.

Financial Data. Proprietary hospitals expended nearly $230 million in 1956, or about $18.90 per patient day. Payroll expenses totaled more than $123 million and the payroll component of total expenses was approximately 53.5 per cent. Total assets in the same period were estimated at close to $217 million, or around $4300 per bed. Almost all operating income is derived from patient revenue. Capital funds come from operating reserves, from loans obtained from banks and other commercial lending agencies, and from the personal resources of the owners of the hospitals.

Educational Activities. Most of the proprietary hospitals are not large enough to support medical and/or nursing education programs. As a result, only nine such hospitals, less than 1 per cent of the total, were approved for internships by the American Medical Association in 1956. Twenty-five, or just over 2 per cent, of the hospitals were approved for residency training. Although completely accurate information is not available, it is estimated that roughly 1.5 per cent of the proprietary hospitals operated approved professional nursing schools and approximately 3 per cent had approved practical nursing programs.

Administration. Proprietary hospitals are usually administered by their owners, who, in most instances, are members of the medical profession. Some of the larger proprietary hospitals have a nonmedical administrator who is hired by and reports to the owners or — in the case of a corporation with a large number of stockholders — the board of directors representing the owners.

Medical Staff. The medical staffs in several of the larger proprietary hospitals are organized by clinical services. However, such a formal organization is not possible in most proprietary institutions as they are usually staffed by only one or two physicians.

Trends. Proprietary hospitals are not only required to pay taxes on their earned income but must also provide the owners with a reasonable return on their investment. Consequently, proprietary hospitals find it difficult to survive in areas where they must compete, both in their rates and in the quality of service they render, with other types of hospitals. In addition, the tremendous amount of capital necessary to build a modern hospital is seldom available to physicians or laymen who might otherwise be interested in hospital development. However, this pattern has a strong appeal for investors seeking the benefits of capital gains. In areas where voluntary efforts move too slowly to meet the community's need for hospital service, the proprietary pattern will prove more efficient and will flourish.

As a result of the above, the steady decline in the number of proprietary hospitals during the past twenty years can reasonably be expected to continue in some areas but will be interrupted sporadically by construction of small institutions in other parts of the country.

Nonprofit Hospitals: Church Affiliated

HOSPITALS owned and/or operated by religious orders of the Roman Catholic Church constitute one of the most important single patterns of ownership and control in the United States. The tremendous effect these institutions have on the entire hospital industry is best illustrated by the following:

1. In 1956 the 874 Roman Catholic hospitals in the continental limits of the United States represented more than 72 per cent of all church owned, operated, or related hospitals; almost 25 per cent of the non-profit hospitals; about 18.5 per cent of the nongovernmental hospitals; and approximately 12.5 per cent of all hospitals in the nation.

2. Roman Catholic hospitals in the same year contained nearly 78 per cent of the beds in church hospitals; over 31 per cent of the non-profit hospital beds; around 28 per cent of the beds in nongovernmental hospitals; and close to 8.6 per cent of all hospital beds in this country.

3. During 1956, Roman Catholic hospitals accounted for more than 81 per cent of all admissions to church hospitals; over 34 per cent of the nonprofit hospital admissions; approximately 31 per cent of all nongovernmental hospital admissions; and almost 23 per cent of the admissions to all hospitals in the United States. In other words, during that year, *nearly one of every four patients entering a hospital in this country was admitted to a Roman Catholic institution.*

4. Over one fourth of the state-approved schools of professional nursing in 1956 were operated by or affiliated with Roman Catholic hospitals.

Organizational Structure and Governing Authority. Almost all hospitals which are known as Roman Catholic institutions are both owned and operated by religious orders. A few Roman Catholic hospitals — less than 4 per cent of the total number in the United States in 1956 — have been turned over to religious orders to operate and manage but are owned by other church bodies, industrial enterprises, voluntary non-profit associations, or governmental units or agencies.

Roman Catholic religious orders are communities of men or women bound together within the Church by the vows of poverty, chastity, and obedience. Most religious orders are expected to be self-sufficient and are relatively independent of each other and of other Roman Catholic organizations; however, *all* orders must abide by the canon laws of the Church.

There were more than 300 Roman Catholic religious orders in the United States in 1956 and approximately 180 of these orders owned and/or operated hospitals. Of the latter group, all but three were sisterhoods. Many sisterhoods control just one hospital while others own and/or operate a large number of such institutions.

Most sisterhoods are organized in a similar manner. Typically, they are headed by a religious superior known as the Mother General, have a central office or headquarters called the generalate, and are governed by a generalate council of which the Mother General and Assistant Mother General are members. Many of the sisterhoods are quite large and are divided into geographic areas called provinces. These areas are governed by provincial councils and are headed by a religious superior known as the Mother Provincial.

The following order is fairly representative of sisterhoods which own and operate a number of hospitals and a discussion of its organizational structure is presented to provide a better understanding of the Roman Catholic pattern of hospital ownership and control.

The Sisters of St. Joseph of Carondelet. Founded in Le Puy, France, in 1650, the Sisters of St. Joseph of Carondelet currently own and operate fourteen hospitals in ten states (Arizona, California, Georgia, Idaho, Michigan, Minnesota, Missouri, New York, North Dakota, and Washington). The order is divided geographically into five provinces and has its generalate in St. Louis, Missouri.

Governing the affairs of the sisterhood is a generalate council of five members — including the Mother General and the Assistant Mother General — each of whom represents one of the five provinces. The Mother General, her assistant, and the other three council members are elected to their positions by the general chapter, which convenes every six years and includes four representatives from each province: the Mother Provincial and three delegates elected directly by the sisters of the province. Generalate council members, including the Mother General and her assistant, serve six-year terms and may be re-elected once. The council meets monthly and all members reside at the mother house in St. Louis during their term of office.

The provinces are governed by provincial councils patterned after the generalate council. Each provincial council meets monthly and has five members: the Mother Provincial and Assistant Provincial, who are appointed by the generalate council, and three other members who are appointed by the Mother Provincial. All provincial council members, including the Mother Provincial and her assistant, serve three-year terms and may be reappointed once.

Each hospital within a particular province has its own governing board which, again, is composed of five members. The Mother Provincial and Assistant Provincial serve as the president and vice-president, respectively, of the governing board of *every* hospital within the province. The three remaining members of an individual hospital's governing board are elected each year by the governing board itself from among the sisters in the hospital and may be re-elected indefinitely. Although every sister in the hospital is eligible for board membership, the administrator and assistant administrator are almost always elected to fill two of the vacancies. The business office manager frequently is selected as the third member. The governing board of a hospital is required to meet once annually and other meetings are scheduled as needed. The three board members from within the hospital, of course, live and work together and meet informally on many occasions.

Lay Advisory Boards. A fairly recent development in many, but not all, Roman Catholic hospitals is the creation of lay advisory boards. Such a board usually consists of from ten to fifteen members who — in an attempt to get a cross-section of the community in which the hospital is located — represent business and civic groups, industry, labor, management, different religions, and a variety of nationalities. Lay advisory boards generally hold monthly meetings. As their name implies, these boards serve strictly in an advisory capacity and have no authority over hospital operation. Nevertheless, if utilized properly, they are of invaluable assistance to the administrators and governing boards of Roman Catholic hospitals.

Diocesan Hospital Directors. The bishop in a diocese containing one or more Roman Catholic hospitals usually appoints one of the priests in the diocese to act as the diocesan hospital director. The functions and duties of these hospital directors apparently vary a great deal from one diocese to another and depend, to a large degree, on the hospital director's background and training and on the customs and traditions in the different dioceses. Normally, a diocesan hospital director has no authority over Roman Catholic hospitals. However, he may advise and consult with the administrators and governing boards of the hospitals in his diocese on certain problems. In addition, he frequently represents the Roman Catholic hospitals in his diocese at civic, professional, and religious functions and often serves as a liaison between these hospitals, the bishop, and the community.

History of Growth and Development. In 1524 the Spanish conqueror Cortez built the Hospital of the Immaculate Conception in Mexico City and entrusted its operation to a Roman Catholic nursing brotherhood. Now known as the Hospital of Jesus of Nazareth, it is the oldest hospital on the North American continent with a continuous history of service.

De Paul Hospital in St. Louis, Missouri, is the oldest existing Roman Catholic hospital in the United States and was the first hospital of any type west of the Mississippi River. Originally called the St. Louis Hospital, it was founded in 1828 by the Daughters of St. Vincent de Paul.

St. Joseph Infirmary in Louisville, Kentucky, was established in 1836 by the Sisters of Charity of Nazareth and, in 1840, the hospital which is now known as Mount Hope Retreat opened in Baltimore, Maryland.

Of the total number of Roman Catholic hospitals in operation in this country in 1956, nearly one third were already in existence at the turn of the century and more than one half were established in the period from 1900 to 1945. Approximately 17 per cent of the Roman Catholic hospitals in 1956 were founded after World War II.

Measures of Significance. The 874 Roman Catholic hospitals in the United States in 1956 had a combined capacity of 137,628 beds. There were nearly five million admissions to these institutions during the year, or more than 36 admissions per bed. The average daily census was estimated at 104,000 patients; the average occupancy rate exceeded 75 per cent.

Of these 874 institutions, 830 were short-term hospitals and forty-four provided long-term care. The short-term institutions included 810 general-acute, seventeen maternal, and three pediatric hospitals. Among the long-term facilities were a leprosarium and one cardiac, eleven chronic, two convalescent, two incurable, one mentally deficient, three orthopedic, fourteen psychiatric, and nine tuberculosis hospitals.

Over 76 per cent of the hospitals were accredited by the Joint Commission on Accreditation of Hospitals. Completely valid data were not available on the number of continental Roman Catholic hospitals that belonged to the American Hospital Association and state and/or regional associations; however, the vast majority of Roman Catholic hospitals were believed to be members of these groups.

Roman Catholic hospitals are generally quite large. In 1956 their average capacity exceeded 157 beds. Nearly 40 per cent of the institutions had less than 100 beds and about 13 per cent contained 300 beds or more. At the extremes, only 3.2 per cent of the hospitals had fewer than 25 beds and under 2 per cent had a capacity above 500 beds.

Patterns of Hospital Ownership and Control

Roman Catholic hospitals are widely scattered throughout the United States and every state in the union has at least one such institution. The most dense concentration is in the midwest in the American Hospital Association's East North Central and West North Central regions which together contain almost one half of the Roman Catholic hospitals in this country. They are most sparsely distributed in the East South Central, New England, and South Atlantic regions. Among the individual states, Illinois had seventy-one Roman Catholic hospitals in 1956 while only one such hospital was located in Delaware.

Personnel. In 1956 approximately 209,000 persons were estimated to be employed in Roman Catholic hospitals, or 2.02 employees per patient.

Although they hold most of the key positions, members of a religious order generally account for only a small proportion of total hospital employees. A Roman Catholic hospital in an urban center may have as few as 5 per cent of its personnel who are sisters or brothers. In rural areas, a larger proportion of employees normally are members of religious orders because of the shortage of lay personnel in such areas.

The religious who are employed in a hospital operated, for example, by a sisterhood are generally assigned to a particular department or position by the Mother Provincial or a designated higher superior, not by the hospital administrator. The administrator may recommend sisters to fill certain positions within the hospital or to be withdrawn from jobs for which they are not suited. The final decision, however, rests with the higher superior, who, after careful consideration, may accept or reject such suggestions.

Financial Data. The total assets of Roman Catholic hospitals in the United States in 1956 were estimated to exceed $1.6 billion, or roughly $11,800 per bed. Total expenses in the same year were estimated at $950 million, about $25.10 per patient day. Payroll expenses exceeded $496 million and the payroll component of total expenses was approximately 52 per cent.

Members of religious orders who are employed in Roman Catholic hospitals do not receive salaries as such; however, the above payroll and, consequently, total expense figures include amounts for the services of the sisters and brothers which are comparable with the salaries that lay personnel would receive in similar positions.

As stated previously, religious orders and the hospitals they own and operate are expected to be self-sufficient. Therefore, the hospitals do not rely on the dioceses or archdioceses in which they are located or on any other church body for financial assistance. Almost all operating income is derived from patient revenue. Capital funds come from operating reserves, community campaigns, endowments, Hill-Burton grants, and from the religious orders themselves. Normally, a hospital must have the approval of the bishop of the diocese in which it is contained before conducting a community fund campaign.

Educational Activities. Over 27 per cent of the Roman Catholic hospitals in the United States were approved for internships in 1956 by the American Medical Association and nearly 24 per cent were approved for residencies. In addition, fifty-four of the hospitals were affiliated with medical schools.

Educationally, however, Roman Catholic hospitals have their greatest significance in the area of nursing education. Approximately 32 per cent of the hospitals operated professional nursing schools in 1956 and more than 5 per cent were affiliated with collegiate schools of basic nursing. As previously mentioned, over one fourth of the state-approved schools of professional nursing during that year were operated by or affiliated with Roman Catholic hospitals. In addition to the professional nursing programs, about 4 per cent of the Roman Catholic hospitals had schools for practical nurses.

The various Roman Catholic hospitals also offer courses in medical record library science, medical technology, X-ray technology, dietetics, social service, physical therapy, occupational therapy, and other paramedical fields.

Administration. A Roman Catholic hospital is almost always administered by a member of the religious order which owns and operates the institution. In the case of a hospital controlled by a sisterhood, the sister-administrator is normally appointed by the Mother General and is responsible to her Mother Provincial or a designated higher superior.

Every Roman Catholic hospital has a religious superior whose duties include administering the hospital convent and providing an environment conducive to a spiritual life. As the number of religious in most Roman Catholic hospitals is quite small, the administrator frequently is also the religious superior of the hospital convent. However, the term of a religious superior is limited by canon law, ordinarily to six years of continuous service in one convent. An individual order may, through its constitution and bylaws, limit a religious superior's term of office even further but cannot extend it. The importance of this rule, from an administrative standpoint, is that when the administrator-superior are one, the administration of the hospital changes every six years or less. On the other hand, when the administrator and superior are separate, the administrator's term of office is usually indefinite.

The number of nonmedical administrative personnel in Roman Catholic hospitals appears to be increasing. Nonmedical assistant administrators and administrative assistants are quite commonly employed and a few hospitals have nonmedical administrators.

Medical Staff. The medical staffs in most Roman Catholic hospitals are organized by clinical services under a medical director or chief of staff. Qualifications for staff membership are similar to those in other nonprofit, nongovernmental hospitals. The medical staff bylaws must of course be observed by all staff physicians, and such bylaws reflect certain teachings of the Church in regard to the procedures permitted or restricted.

The Catholic Hospital Association of the United States and Canada. Established in 1915, the Catholic Hospital Association of the United States and Canada is currently composed of approximately 1400 hospitals and related institutions. The association has its headquarters in St. Louis, Missouri, and is organized and operates along the same lines as the American Hospital Association. It holds an annual convention, publishes a monthly journal and an annual directory, and provides consultation services. It also sponsors a significant number of educational institutes and seminars each year.

Other Associations of Roman Catholic Hospitals. In addition to the national association there were thirty-four Roman Catholic hospital conferences in the United States in 1956, organized on regional, state, diocesan, and local levels. Most of these conferences hold regular meetings and have their own constitution and bylaws while a few function only on an informal basis.

Trends. Roman Catholic hospital and health facilities in the United States have increased significantly in recent years. In the period from 1952 through 1956 fifty-four new hospitals were established, with a total capacity of nearly 4500 beds. In addition, thirty-five other hospitals were nearing completion or were in the process of being developed. In the future, Roman Catholic hospitals should continue to increase in number as the population grows and as finances remain in voluntary control.

LUTHERAN HOSPITALS

Located throughout the country, but particularly in rural communities in the midwestern and mountain states, are a large number of Lutheran hospitals which provide hospitalization in a spiritual setting to more than one third of a million patients annually. These institutions accounted for approximately 11 per cent of all church-operated or related hospitals in the United States in 1956 and for almost one third of all Protestant hospitals in the nation.

Organizational Structure and Governing Authority. Lutheran hospitals exhibit many different ownership and control patterns. Some of the hospitals are both owned and controlled by a national Lutheran Church body or by one of its jurisdictional units or segments. Other Lutheran hospitals are owned by an independent corporation but are controlled by a particular Lutheran synod or by a group of Lutheran churches in a certain area. Some of the hospitals are both owned and controlled independently, but are recognized as Lutheran institutions by one of the national church bodies. Still other Lutheran hospitals are neither owned nor recognized by a national church body or by a group of churches, but simply consider themselves to be Lutheran institutions or, through tradition, are considered as such by the general public.

Most Lutheran hospitals have a separate board of trustees. However, some hospitals are governed by the boards of the national church bodies, which own and/or control them.

History of Growth and Development. The development of Lutheran hospitals in the United States, as well as the growth of hospitals among other Protestant denominations, was greatly influenced by the deaconess movement, initiated by Pastor Theodore Fliedner and his wife Fredricke, in Kaiserswerth, Germany. The Fliedners established the first deaconess hospital and the first school for deaconess nurses in 1836. Ten years later, the Reverend Dr. William A. Passavant, pastor of an English Lutheran church in Pittsburgh, Pennsylvania, visited Kaiserswerth and was so impressed with the services of the deaconesses that he made plans to introduce the same system in the United States. In 1849 Dr. Passavant, with the help of four deaconesses sent from Germany by Pastor Fliedner, established a deaconess hospital in Pittsburgh. Presently named for its founder, Passavant Hospital is not only the oldest Lutheran hospital in the United States, but is also the oldest Protestant hospital in this country.

The success of the Pittsburgh hospital led to the development of other Lutheran deaconess hospitals in the latter part of the nineteenth century and spurred other Protestant groups, such as the Methodists and Episcopalians, to establish deaconess societies and hospitals of their own.

Fifteen, or nearly 13 per cent, of the Lutheran hospitals in operation in 1956 had been founded by the turn of the century. From 1900 to 1930, Lutheran hospitals gradually but steadily increased in number. Their rate of growth dropped significantly during the depression years of the 1930s and the war years of the 1940s. However, with the end of World War II, they began to increase rapidly, and more than one half of the Lutheran hospitals currently in operation have been established since 1945.

Measures of Significance. There were 135 known Lutheran hospitals in the United States in 1956, with an estimated combined capacity of 11,200 beds. During the year nearly 389,000 patients were admitted to these institutions, or approximately 35 admissions per bed. The average

103

daily census in the same period was about 7900 patients; the average occupancy rate exceeded 70.5 per cent.

All but seven of these Lutheran hospitals were general-acute facilities. The seven "special" hospitals included a college infirmary, an orthopedic hospital, a psychiatric institution, two chronic disease and convalescent facilities, and two tuberculosis hospitals.

Around 72 per cent of the hospitals were members of the American Hospital Association, and almost 94 per cent belonged to state and/or regional associations. Less than 38 per cent were accredited by the Joint Commission on Accreditation of Hospitals.

Lutheran hospitals are typically quite small. Their average capacity was under 85 beds in 1956 and nearly 55 per cent of the hospitals had less than 50 beds. Only five Lutheran hospitals contained 300 beds or more. The 13-bed infirmary at St. Olaf College in Northfield, Minnesota, was the smallest Lutheran hospital. The largest was Emanuel Hospital in Portland, Oregon, with 431 beds.

Over 16,000 persons were employed in Lutheran hospitals in 1956, or approximately 2.03 employees per patient.

Lutheran hospitals are naturally concentrated in areas which have a large Lutheran population. Almost 84 per cent of these institutions in 1956 were located west of the Mississippi River, particularly in the American Hospital Association's West North Central and Mountain regions, which had seventy-nine and twenty-four Lutheran hospitals respectively. Kansas and North Dakota both contained eighteen Lutheran hospitals, and Nebraska had seventeen such institutions. In North Dakota, Lutheran hospitals accounted for nearly 29 per cent of all the hospitals in the state.

Financial Data. Lutheran hospitals expended an estimated $69.5 million in 1956, or roughly $24.10 per patient day. Payroll expenses in the same period were estimated at nearly $42 million and the payroll component of total expenses was approximately 60.4 per cent. Total assets were evaluated at more than $104 million, or around $9300 per bed.

Patient revenue is the principal source of operating income. Capital funds are derived from operating reserves, community campaigns, Hill-Burton grants, endowments, gifts from Lutheran church bodies and congregations, and loans from banks and other commercial sources.

Educational Activities. Most Lutheran hospitals are too small to actively support medical and nursing education programs. Only 12 per cent of the hospitals had been approved for residencies by the American Medical Association in 1956, and less than 17 per cent offered approved internships. Twenty-one per cent of the hospitals operated approved professional nursing schools. Two Lutheran hospitals were affiliated with medical schools, and two had approved practical nurse training programs.

Administration. The administrators of Lutheran hospitals are normally responsible to the boards governing their respective institutions. Most of the hospitals are run by nonmedical administrators and a few are administrated by clergymen.

Medical Staff. Qualifications for medical staff membership in a Lutheran hospital are no different than those imposed by most other nonprofit, nongovernmental hospitals. The medical staffs in the larger hospitals are organized by clinical services under a medical director or chief of staff. However, in the majority of Lutheran hospitals, the staffs are too small to be organized in such a manner.

Lutheran Hospitals and Homes Society of America, Inc. The Lutheran Hospitals and Homes Society is a nonprofit organization which, in 1956, owned and/or operated fifty-nine institutions — including fifty-one hospitals — in the states of Colorado, Kansas, Montana, Nebraska, North Dakota, South Dakota, Wisconsin, and Wyoming. The society has its central offices in Fargo, North Dakota, and is incorporated under the laws of that state.

The society was formed in 1938 by a group of Lutheran ministers and laymen, who felt the responsibility, as Christian men and women, of making a contribution to the care of the distressed. Voting membership was and is limited by the society's constitution and bylaws to persons who have a formal affiliation with a Lutheran church. However, at no time in its existence has the society been subsidized by any church or church group or by any other agency. The society is, and always has been, a separate and individual corporate entity.

The society is governed by a board of not less than nine nor more than twenty-one directors, who are elected by the voting members from among their ranks. One third of the directors are elected for three-year terms at each annual meeting of the society.

The society performs the following functions for communities in the areas it serves and for the hospitals it owns and operates: (1) analyzes the hospital needs of communities; (2) assists communities in financing hospitals; (3) plans hospital buildings; (4) supervises the administration of hospitals; (5) formulates operating policies and standards; (6) reduces the cost of hospital operations through centralized accounting and purchasing; (7) recruits personnel; (8) develops uniform records and reports; (9) supervises and approves hospital insurance programs.

Trends. As stated previously, more than one half of the present Lutheran hospitals have opened since the end of World War II. In the future, the number of Lutheran hospitals and beds should continue to increase slowly, dependent upon the location of population and upon the availability of voluntary funds to finance capital construction.

METHODIST HOSPITALS

The Methodist Church feels the religious motive is still inherent in the "voluntary" system of providing hospital care and that both the motive and the system must be preserved. To meet this challenge and the additional challenge posed by the ever-increasing demand for hospital and health services, there were seventy-two Methodist hospitals in the United States in 1956 and more were in the process of development.

Organizational Structure and Governing Authority. The Methodist Church is divided, for administrative purposes, into Annual Conferences. At present, there are ninety-six such conferences in the United States.

Each Methodist hospital is owned, operated, and maintained by a separate corporation and has its own board of trustees. However, in most cases, the individual Annual Conferences exert control over the Methodist hospitals within their jurisdictions by electing the members of the hospitals' boards of trustees.

Only a few Methodist hospitals are not controlled in this manner by an Annual Conference. These hospitals were founded by a society of the Methodist Church which is no longer in existence. Nevertheless, they can continue to be known as Methodist institutions because at least 75 per cent of the members of the boards of trustees are Methodists.

The governing boards of the hospitals controlled by the Annual Conferences are usually quite large with thirty-five to fifty members. Such a board normally has an executive committee, composed of ten to fifteen board members, which is empowered to act for the trustees in the interim between board meetings.

History of Growth and Development. The Methodist religion is the outgrowth of a small religious club formed in 1729, at Oxford University in England, by John and Charles Wesley and others. Shortly after the formation of this club, John Wesley established a dispensary in the Old Foundry in London. This was the first Methodist institution for the care of the sick, and initiated the present work of the Methodist Church in the hospital field.

The Methodist Hospital of Brooklyn, established in 1881 and still in operation, was apparently the first Methodist hospital in the United States. The Good Shepherd Hospital of Syracuse University was founded nine years earlier, in 1872, but presumably was not a Methodist institution when originally opened.

106

Nonprofit Hospitals: Church Affiliated

Over 26 per cent of the Methodist hospitals in operation in 1956 were established before the turn of the century. Twenty-four hospitals were founded during the 1920s while only ten hospitals have opened since 1931.

Measures of Significance. In 1956 the seventy-two Methodist hospitals (all were general-acute institutions) had a reported capacity of 16,085 beds. There were 705,522 admissions to these hospitals during the year, or nearly 44 admissions per bed. The average daily census was 12,658 patients; the average occupancy rate was about 79 per cent.

The hospitals ranged in size from two 38-bed institutions — Boothroy Memorial Hospital in Goodland, Kansas, and Kenmare Deaconess Hospital in Kenmare, North Dakota — to the 1062-bed Barnes Hospital in St. Louis, Missouri. The average capacity exceeded 223 beds and one third of the hospitals contained 300 beds or more.

Approximately 89 per cent of the hospitals were accredited by the Joint Commission on Accreditation of Hospitals. All seventy-two hospitals were members of state and/or regional hospital associations and all but one belonged to the American Hospital Association.

In 1956 over 29,000 persons were employed in Methodist hospitals, or roughly 2.32 employees per patient. Nearly three fourths of the hospitals employed a chaplain on either a full- or part-time basis.

The seventy-two Methodist hospitals were not well distributed throughout the United States, even though all of the American Hospital Association's geographic regions contained at least one such institution. They were concentrated in the Midwest, particularly in the East North Central and West North Central regions, which together contained forty Methodist hospitals, or almost 56 per cent of the total.

Financial Data. The seventy-two hospitals reportedly expended $120,706,000 in 1956, or more than $26.00 per patient day. Payroll expense figures for the same year were not available, but were estimated at about $75 million. Total assets of Methodist Hospitals exceeded $231 million, or close to $14,400 per bed.

Patient revenue is the principal source of operating income. In addition, more than one third of the Annual Conferences have "Golden Cross" societies which raise funds for Methodist hospitals and homes through an annual enrollment in the various Methodist congregations. The respective conferences direct the use of such funds and, consequently, money raised in this manner apparently may be used for different purposes. However, in many conferences, Golden Cross funds are used to provide "free service" in the hospitals and homes.

Capital funds for construction and expansion come from operating reserves, community campaigns, grants from foundations and the federal government, endowments, and loans from banks and other commercial sources.

Educational Activities. As a group, Methodist hospitals were extremely active in the area of education in 1956. Thirty-four hospitals were approved by the American Medical Association for internships and the same number had been approved for residency training. Eight hospitals were affiliated with medical schools. In addition, fifty-two hospitals, or over 72 per cent of the total, operated professional nursing schools and seven hospitals had practical nursing programs. In 1956 nearly 7000 nursing students were in training in Methodist hospitals.

Administration. The administrators of Methodist hospitals report directly to their respective boards of trustees. The majority of the administrators are nonmedical individuals; however, physicians are in charge of several hospitals, and more than 20 per cent of the hospitals in 1956 were administered by doctors of divinity and theology.

Medical Staff. The medical staffs in most of the hospitals are large enough to be organized by clinical services under a medical director or chief of staff. Such an organization is not possible in some of the smaller hospitals because the staffs are too limited in size.

The Board of Hospitals and Homes of the Methodist Church. The Board of Hospitals and Homes is the official agency of the Methodist Church in the fields of health and welfare. According to the board's constitution, "hospitals or homes known as institutions of The Methodist Church . . . or looking to the Methodist constituency for support . . . shall be expected to affiliate with the Board of Hospitals and Homes." Emphasis must be placed on the word "affiliate" as the Board of Hospitals and Homes does not own or operate any of the institutions associated with it. Its primary functions are to advise the various hospitals and homes and to assist them in meeting their objectives. In 1956, 207 institutions — seventy-two hospitals, eighty homes for older persons, forty-three homes for children, seven homes for business women, and five special agencies including two homes for unwed mothers — were affiliated with the Board of Hospitals and Homes. The board assists these institutions by (1) making surveys; (2) formulating standards; (3) disseminating information; (4) suggesting fund-raising plans; (5) providing architectural data; (6) maintaining a personnel service; (7) strengthening institutional-church relationships; (8) providing consultation on all forms of operation in its affiliated institutions including nursing service and nursing education.

The board also renders assistance, other than financial, in the establishment of new institutions and is empowered to act as trustee for the administration of bequests and endowments. The board is not responsible, either legally or morally, for the debts, contracts, or obligations of the institutions affiliated with it.

Control of the Board of Hospitals and Homes is vested in an eighteen-man Board of Managers composed of two bishops; one minister and one layman from each of six Jurisdictional Conferences; and four members-at-large. The two bishops are elected by the Council of Bishops. The representatives from the Jurisdictional Conferences, which are geographic divisions of the Methodist Church, are selected by the conferences themselves, and at least one of the two from each conference must be the active administrator of an institution affiliated with the Board of Hospitals and Homes. The four members-at-large are elected by the Board of Managers itself. All eighteen members serve four-year terms and all are required to be Methodists.

In addition to the national or general Board of Hospitals and Homes, each Annual Conference is required to maintain a Conference Board of Hospitals and Homes to promote, in cooperation with the national board, the interests of the hospitals and other institutions within the jurisdiction of the conference. It is also suggested, though not required, that every Methodist church should have a Committee on Hospitals and Homes to disseminate information, take charge of the annual Golden Cross enrollment, and perform similar functions.

The National Association of Methodist Hospitals and Homes. The National Association of Methodist Hospitals and Homes is composed of "representatives of institutions and presidents of Jurisdictional and Conference Boards connected with Methodist philanthropy." It has its own constitution and bylaws, meets in convention once a year, and operates under the general direction of the Board of Hospitals and Homes. The purpose of the association is to lift the spiritual, scientific, and financial standards of the hospitals and homes of the Methodist Church.

Trends. Several new Methodist hospitals were being developed during 1956 and certainly other hospitals will be added in the future. However, it appears the significance of Methodist hospitals to the entire hospital industry will remain relatively constant in coming years.

PRESBYTERIAN HOSPITALS

The Presbyterian Church feels it has an obligation to minister to the temporal as well as the spiritual needs of men. Among these temporal needs is adequate health care and, in this regard, the obligation felt by the Church is concretely expressed by the Presbyterian hospitals, nursing homes, and outpatient clinics located in the United States and throughout the world.

Organizational Structure and Governing Authority. Hospitals which

109

are known as Presbyterian institutions vary greatly in their ownership and control and in their relationship to the Church. Of the twenty Presbyterian hospitals in operation in this country in 1957, five were directly owned and operated; two were operated by boards which were *controlled* by jurisdictional bodies of the Church; eight were operated by boards *related* to such jurisdictional bodies; two were operated by boards related to groups of churches or to other Presbyterian organizations; three were independent.

All but one of the institutions in the first group were directly owned and operated by the Board of National Missions. The lone exception — Abbott Hospital in Minneapolis, Minnesota — has a particularly unique organizational structure and will be subsequently discussed in greater detail.

Most of the hospitals fell into the third category. Their governing boards were either nominated by, or approved by, or reported to, or had some relationship with a synod, presbytery, or local church.

All of the three so-called independent hospitals enjoyed some kind of relationship with the Church but were not legally tied to it or to any of its agencies.

Abbott Hospital, Minneapolis, Minnesota. So far as is known, Abbott Hospital is the only hospital in the United States which is both owned and operated by a single church congregation. A service of the Westminster Presbyterian Church of Minneapolis, the hospital is technically governed by the church's board of trustees. In actual practice, however, the responsibility for hospital operation is vested in a committee of the board appointed for that specific purpose. Although the actions and recommendations of this hospital committee must be formally approved by the entire church board, such approval is almost automatic.

The hospital is not incorporated. The church is the corporate body, and its seal is affixed to any hospital documents requiring such authentication. All endowments to the hospital are also handled by the church.

History. In 1803 a group calling themselves "friends of humanity" sent 250 copies of a publication describing a new method of smallpox vaccination to the General Assembly of the Presbyterian Church with the request that they be sent "by the missionaries from this Assembly to the frontiers of the country and distributed for the caution and direction of those who have less opportunity of obtaining medical aid and advice." The interest of the Presbyterian Church in the field of public health stems from the Assembly's compliance with this request.

Shortly thereafter, a committee of the Church sent a supply of vaccines and other medicines to a school for Cherokee Indians. Later on, medical service became an established part of the missionary program of the Church.

110

Outside of the missionary program, the concern of the Church for hospital development found concrete expression in a number of cities. Harper Hospital was established in Detroit in 1863, and Presbyterian Hospital in New York City was founded in 1868. Other Presbyterian hospitals were developed in Philadelphia, Baltimore, Chicago, and Pittsburgh before the end of the nineteenth century, and five additional hospitals were established in the first ten years of the twentieth century. The most recent addition is the Presbyterian Intercommunity Hospital in Whittier, California, founded in 1959.

Measures of Significance. The twenty Presbyterian hospitals in operation within the continental limits of the United States in 1957 had a combined capacity in excess of 5300 beds. There were nearly 174,000 admissions to these institutions during that year, or roughly 33 admissions per bed. The average daily census was approximately 4360 patients; the average occupancy rate was over 80 per cent.

All twenty hospitals were short-term institutions. Nineteen provided care of a general nature while one specialized in the treatment of patients with eye, ear, nose, and throat diseases.

The average capacity of the Presbyterian hospitals was around 265 beds. Seven hospitals had less than 100 beds and only two hospitals had over 500 beds. They ranged in size from the 17-bed Jane Cook Hospital in Frenchburg, Kentucky, to the 1516-bed Presbyterian Hospital in New York City.

Sixteen of the twenty hospitals were accredited by the Joint Commission on Accreditation of Hospitals in 1957. Nineteen of the institutions were members of the American Hospital Association and seventeen belonged to state or regional associations.

More than 11,000 persons were employed in Presbyterian hospitals during the same period, or approximately 2.6 employees per patient.

Geographically, Presbyterian hospitals were almost evenly divided east and west of the Mississippi River in 1957 and were located in seven of the nine American Hospital Association regions. Only the New England and West South Central regions had no such institutions.

Financial Data. Presbyterian hospitals expended over $54 million in 1957, or roughly $34.00 per patient day. Payroll expenses in the same period were estimated at $33 million, nearly 61 per cent of the total expenditures. Total assets of the twenty institutions were estimated to be in excess of $150 million, or more than $28,000 per bed.

Operating income is derived almost exclusively from fees for services rendered. Capital funds come from a variety of sources: operating reserves, Hill-Burton grants, community campaigns, and commercial loans.

Educational Activities. As a group, Presbyterian hospitals are quite active in the area of education. This is evidenced by the fact that in 1957

111

ten such hospitals — 50 per cent of the total — were approved by the American Medical Association for residencies, and a similar number had internship approval. Four hospitals also maintained medical school affiliations. In addition, nine of the twenty institutions operated approved professional nursing schools and four others were affiliated with such schools.

Administration. The administration of Presbyterian hospitals is similar to that of other voluntary, nonprofit hospital patterns. The administrator is normally responsible to a board of trustees or directors for the operation of the institution and coordinates his or her functions with the medical director or chief of staff. In 1957 the management of some Presbyterian hospitals was entrusted to physicians; however, the majority were being administered by nonmedical people.

Medical Staff. The organization of the Presbyterian hospital medical staffs also follows that of other voluntary, nonprofit patterns. In the larger institutions the staff is divided into clinical services, each of which is headed by a chief. The activities of the various chiefs are coordinated by a medical director or a chief of staff who is also responsible for the hospital's over-all medical care program.

Trends. Some expansion in the number of Presbyterian hospitals and hospital beds will certainly occur in future years. However, it is anticipated that this expansion will be a gradual process and that the significance of Presbyterian hospitals to the total hospital industry will remain relatively unchanged.

BAPTIST HOSPITALS

Forty-four hospitals — six in the northern part of the United States and thirty-eight in the south — were known to be owned and/or controlled by or related, in some manner, to the Baptist churches and their various jurisdictional and state conventions in 1956.

Organizational Structure and Governing Authority. The Baptist hospitals in the north are all owned and controlled by separate corporations. Each corporation is governed by a board of trustees of which the majority of members must usually be Baptists.

Almost all southern Baptist hospitals are apparently both owned and controlled by the Baptist convention of the state in which they are located. Such a hospital has its own board of trustees, appointed by its respective state convention. Once the board members are appointed, the state convention generally does not interfere with their trusteeship and they are relatively free to run the hospital as they see fit in meeting the needs of their particular community.

History of Growth and Development. Only two of the present Baptist hospitals were established prior to 1900. The Missouri Baptist Hospital in St. Louis opened in 1884, and the New England Baptist Hospital in Boston, Massachusetts, was founded in 1893. Fifty per cent of the Baptist hospitals in operation in 1956 were established in the period from 1900 to 1930, and nearly 32 per cent had opened since the end of World War II.

Measures of Significance. In 1956 the forty-four known Baptist hospitals in the United States had a total capacity of 9318 beds. There were an estimated 388,000 admissions to these beds during the year, or approximately 42 admissions per bed. The average daily census in the same period was estimated at 6949 patients; the average occupancy rate was almost 75 per cent.

The forty-four hospitals — all general-acute institutions — were typically quite large, with an average capacity of nearly 212 beds. They ranged in size from the 12-bed G. L. Prince Hospital in Crockett, Texas, to the 722-bed Baptist Memorial Hospital in Memphis, Tennessee. Twenty-five per cent of the hospitals had less than 100 beds and 25 per cent contained 300 beds or more.

Approximately 80 per cent of the Baptist hospitals were accredited by the Joint Commission on Accreditation of Hospitals in 1956. More than 93 per cent were members of the American Hospital Association and nearly 98 per cent belonged to state and/or regional hospital associations.

Over 16,000 persons were employed in the Baptist hospitals, or roughly 2.4 employees per patient.

The forty-four hospitals were located in seven of the nine American Hospital Association geographic regions. However, they were concentrated in the three southern regions — the South Atlantic, East South Central, and West South Central — which together contained more than 86 per cent of all the Baptist hospitals in the United States. There were no Baptist hospitals in the Mountain or Pacific regions.

Financial Data. In 1956 the forty-four known Baptist hospitals expended an estimated $62,457,000, or approximately $24.60 per patient day. Payroll expenses in the same period totaled nearly $36 million. The payroll component of total expenses was about 58 per cent. Total assets in 1956 were evaluated at nearly $99 million, or around $10,600 per bed.

Almost all operating income is derived from patient revenues. Funds for new construction, expansion, and capital improvements are principally obtained from operating reserves, Hill-Burton grants, community campaigns, and gifts from individuals and the various Baptist churches.

Educational Activities. The typical Baptist hospital is large enough to support medical and nursing education programs. As a group, Baptist hospitals are extremely active in these areas.

The American Medical Association had approved over one third of

113

the hospitals for residency training in 1956 and more than 27 per cent were approved for internships. Three hospitals were affiliated with medical schools. Nearly 55 per cent of the hospitals operated approved professional nursing schools, and five hospitals had approved practical nursing programs.

Administration. Each Baptist hospital administrator is appointed by his respective institution's board of trustees. He coordinates his functions with the medical director or chief of staff and is responsible to the board for the operation of the hospital. At least 14 per cent of the hospitals are administered by clergymen.

Medical Staff. Most Baptist hospital medical staffs are organized by clinical services under a medical director or chief of staff. Such a formal medical staff organization is not possible in some of the smaller hospitals because of the limited number of staff members.

Association of Baptist Homes and Hospitals. In 1956 the Association of Baptist Homes and Hospitals comprised fourteen homes for children, forty-five homes for the aged, six hospitals in the northern part of the United States, and one hospital in Cordova, Alaska. The association's program includes visiting the member institutions and conferring with the various staffs and boards of trustees, the promotion of church support, and the publication of a bimonthly magazine. Its program *does not include* direct financial support of the member institutions.

Southwide Baptist Hospital Association. The Southwide Baptist Hospital Association consists of the Baptist hospitals in the southern part of the United States. At the association's annual meeting, held in conjunction with the American Protestant Hospital Association convention, speakers and discussion groups cover problems of mutual interest and concern. There are no full-time association staff members, and officers are elected annually to conduct the association's business.

Trends. Baptist hospitals have increased considerably in number in the past decade and certainly some additional hospitals will be established in the future. However, the significance of Baptist hospitals to the total hospital industry should remain relatively constant in the coming years.

LATTER-DAY SAINTS HOSPITALS

Among the Protestant denominations engaged in the operation of one or more hospitals is the Church of Jesus Christ of Latter-Day Saints which owns and administers twelve hospitals in the mountain states of Utah, Idaho, and Wyoming.

Organizational Structure and Governing Authority. Administrative control of the hospital program of the Church of Jesus Christ of Latter-Day Saints is vested in two church bodies — the First Presidency and

114

the Presiding Bishopric — and, more immediately, in the governing boards of the individual hospitals.

The Presiding Bishopric consists of three members — the Presiding Bishop, the First Counselor, and the Second Counselor — each of whom serves as chairman of the governing boards of several hospitals. The Presiding Bishop is currently chairman of eight hospital boards. The First and Second Counselors each chair two boards. In conjunction with the Presiding Bishopric, the administrator of the Dr. William H. Groves Hospital presently acts to a degree as a coordinator and staff advisor in the hospital program of the church.

Each hospital is incorporated as a separate entity. The individual boards are composed of from seven to nine members who are local church and community leaders. Vacancies are filled by the board with the approval of the board chairman. The term of appointment is indefinite. A three-man executive committee, selected from within each board, meets twice a month and handles problems that arise during the interim between monthly board meetings.

History of Growth and Development. The first hospital supported by the church was a unit of twelve beds which opened in 1882 in a renovated barn. Mothered by the Relief Society (the women's organization of the church), the hospital provided care principally to obstetric patients. Although it was expanded to fifty beds in 1884, it ceased to operate six years later for lack of patients.

In 1895 Dr. William H. Groves, a dentist, provided $50,000 in his will for the express purpose of building a hospital for the church in Salt Lake City. The church contributed the rest of the necessary funds and, at a cost of $180,000, a 50-bed general hospital was opened in 1905. Named the Dr. William H. Groves Latter-Day Saints Hospital, it is presently the largest hospital operated by the church.

The Thomas D. Dee Memorial Hospital in Ogden, Utah, was turned over to the church in 1912, and the hospital in Logan, Utah, opened in 1914. Three hospitals were added in the 1920s and the remainder have been established since 1939.

Measures of Significance. The twelve hospitals (ten general, one maternity, and one pediatric) had a combined capacity of 1110 beds in 1956 and an additional 307 beds were under construction. During the year, nearly 50,000 patients were admitted to the hospitals, or approximately 45 admissions per bed. The average daily census was 776 patients and the average occupancy rate was around 70 per cent. More than 1800 persons were employed, or about 2.4 employees per patient.

The hospitals ranged in size from two 15-bed institutions in Panguitch, Utah, and Afton, Wyoming, to the 362-bed Dr. William H. Groves Latter-Day Saints Hospital in Salt Lake City. Although the

115

average capacity was over 92 beds, only four of the twelve hospitals had more than 100 beds.

All of the hospitals were members of their respective state hospital associations and ten of the twelve belonged to the American Hospital Association. Seven hospitals had been accredited by the Joint Commission on Accreditation of Hospitals.

Ten of the hospitals were located in Utah, one in Idaho, and one in Wyoming.

Financial Data. In 1956 the hospitals operated by the Church of Jesus Christ of Latter-Day Saints expended over $7,700,000, or roughly $27.00 per patient day. Payroll expenses exceeded $5 million and the payroll component of total expenditures was over 65 per cent. Total assets of the twelve hospitals were estimated at more than $20 million, or approximately $18,000 per bed.

The hospitals operate primarily on income received from patients for services rendered. The church provides some financial assistance in underwriting the hospitals' charity programs and is also the principal source of funds for new construction and capital improvements.

Educational Activities. Three of the hospitals were approved for residencies by the American Medical Association in 1956, and two were approved for internships. In addition, three hospitals were affiliated with medical schools. Four hospitals were affiliated with professional nursing schools and a similar number with practical nursing programs. Some of the hospitals were also maintaining dietetic intern and administrative residency programs and were training X-ray and laboratory technicians and other personnel.

Administration. The operation of each hospital is in the hands of a nonmedical administrator. He coordinates his functions with the chief of the medical staff and is responsible to the governing board.

Medical Staff. The medical staffs in the various hospitals are organized by services in a manner similar to that employed in most of the hospitals in the United States.

Applicants for membership on the medical staff of the Dr. William H. Groves Hospital in Salt Lake City must have completed both a year of internship and a year of residency or its equivalent in addition to the other usual qualifications. The eleven remaining hospitals do not require the year of residency.

Trends. The history of the Latter-Day Saints hospitals has been one of continuing expansion; the construction program underway in 1956 will add another 307 beds to those already in operation. Certainly some additional beds will be needed and constructed in the coming years. However, it seems doubtful that a tremendous increase will ensue in total number of hospitals and beds operated by the church.

□
□ □
□

Other Nonprofit Hospitals

Most of the nonprofit, nongovernmental hospitals in this country are owned and operated, not by church groups or already existing organizations such as fraternal societies or industrial enterprises, but by voluntary associations of public-spirited citizens who are interested in providing hospital care for their community and who are organized solely for that purpose. To distinguish them from other hospitals, institutions of this type are often referred to as "community" hospitals.

Community hospitals represent the largest and most important single pattern of hospital ownership and control and are the backbone of the voluntary, nonprofit hospital system in the United States. Their significance is illustrated by the following:

1. In 1956, community hospitals comprised approximately 57 per cent of the nonprofit hospitals, 42 per cent of the nongovernmental hospitals, and 29 per cent of all hospitals in this country.

2. Community hospitals in the same year contained roughly 51 per cent of the nonprofit hospital beds, 46 per cent of the beds in nongovernmental hospitals, and 14 per cent of all hospital beds in the continental United States.

3. During 1956 these institutions accounted for about 50 per cent of the admissions to nonprofit hospitals, 46 per cent of the nongovernmental hospital admissions, and 34 per cent of the admissions to all hospitals in the United States. In other words, more than one of every three patients entering a hospital in this country in 1956 was admitted to a community hospital.

4. Community hospitals also represented approximately one fourth of all hospital assets, expenses, and personnel in 1956.

Organizational Structure and Governing Authority. As indicated above, community hospitals are governed by voluntary, nonprofit associations or corporations. Membership in such an association is generally

117

open to any interested citizen; the number of members often runs into hundreds and, in some hospital associations, into thousands. Two types of membership, annual and permanent, are usually available, both of which entitle the member to a vote at any meeting of the association or corporation. Annual memberships must be renewed each year and normally are granted upon receipt of a nominal sum, ten dollars or less, which either goes directly to the hospital or is used to defray the costs of operating the hospital association. Permanent memberships are good for life and are generally obtained through the donation of a relatively large amount of money, one hundred dollars or more, to the hospital.

Some community hospitals are operated by hospital corporations set up as nonprofit, joint-stock companies. Both annual and permanent memberships in such a corporation are obtained through the purchase of non-interest-bearing stock, and stock certificates are often issued as evidence of membership.

These voluntary, nonprofit hospital associations and corporations normally meet only once a year. The major, frequently the only, purpose of the annual meeting is to elect new members to the hospital board of trustees or directors. The board has the primary responsibility for the operation of the hospital and is usually composed of from five to fifteen association or corporation members whose terms are staggered so that only one third or one fourth of the board members are elected each year. Normally, the board meets monthly, has its own bylaws, and selects its own officers. It generally maintains certain standing committees—executive, finance, personnel, nursing, public relations, and so on — which have definitely assigned duties of a permanent nature, and it also appoints special committees for temporary tasks.

The executive committee is usually composed of the officers of the board of trustees. It acts for the board in the interval between board meetings. The following examples depict two variations in the organization and control of community hospitals.

Uniontown Hospital, Uniontown, Pennsylvania. Established in 1902, this 280-bed general-acute institution is owned by the Uniontown Hospital Association, a nonprofit association of approximately one hundred representative members of the community. Direct operating control of the hospital is vested in a board of twelve trustees who are elected at the annual meeting of the association from within the membership. They serve three-year terms and may be re-elected indefinitely. The terms are staggered, so that roughly one third of the trustees are elected each year. Board officers (the president, vice president, secretary, and treasurer) are elected annually by the board from among the membership.

The board meets monthly to handle hospital affairs. An executive

118

committee of three trustees, also elected annually by the board, is empowered to act for the board in the interim between board meetings.

The administrator of the hospital is appointed by the board of trustees and is responsible to the board for the management of the institution.

The hospital medical staff is organized by clinical services under the direction of the staff president. He and the other officers are elected by the staff and serve one-year terms. The major clinical services meet monthly, and the entire staff meets four times a year. An executive committee, appointed by the staff president, acts for the medical staff in the interval between the quarterly meetings.

Charles T. Miller Hospital, Inc., St. Paul, Minnesota. This hospital, a 391-bed general-acute institution, differs from many other community hospitals in that no large association is involved in its ownership or operation. The hospital was incorporated in 1916 by five individuals who acted as the first board of directors. The size of the governing board was increased to twenty-one members in 1927 and to thirty members in 1954.

The board is, and always has been, self-perpetuating, and when a director dies or resigns, the remaining directors select a successor. Some of the directors are selected for a specific period of time while others serve indefinitely.

The board has five officers: a chairman, president, first vice president, second vice president, and secretary-treasurer. They are elected annually by the board from among the directors and may be re-elected indefinitely.

The entire board meets only four times a year and the primary responsibility for the operation of the hospital rests with the executive committee which meets monthly. This committee is composed of seven members: the five board officers plus two other directors appointed annually by the board.

Other standing committees maintained by the board are the finance, personnel, facilities, patient care, education and research, community relations, and nominating committees and the joint conference committee on medical affairs. Normally these committees do not hold regular meetings but get together only as required. The members of these committees are appointed by the president of the board, with the approval of the executive committee. Some of the eight committees are composed entirely of board directors plus the administrator of the hospital. Others have directors, key hospital employees, staff physicians, and representatives of the community at large as committee members.

The Charles T. Miller Hospital is primarily a "specialist" institution, and its medical staff is divided into eight clinical services: medicine, surgery, obstetrics and gynecology, neuropsychiatry, ophthalmology, anesthesiology, radiology, and pathology. The chiefs of the services are elected annually by the services themselves.

The officers of the medical staff consist of a president, first vice president, and second vice president. They are elected each year by the staff and may be re-elected once. In actual practice, however, they usually serve just one term. The administration of the hospital provides the services of a secretary and treasurer.

The medical policy board of the Charles T. Miller Hospital functions in a manner similar to the executive committee in the medical staff organization of other hospitals. The board has fifteen members: the chiefs of seven of the eight clinical services, the chairmen of three of the five staff standing committees, the three staff officers, the hospital administrator, and the assistant administrator for medical services.

The five staff standing committees referred to above are the credentials committee, the committee on ancillary medical services, the administrative policy committee, the education and research committee, and the committee on the professional management of patient care. The latter is subdivided into the tissue and medical records committees. The chairmen of these five committees are elected by the membership of the active medical staff. The remaining members are annually appointed by the staff president, with the approval of the medical policy board.

The entire medical staff meets four times a year. The medical policy board and the major clinical services meet monthly.

History of Growth and Development. The voluntary, nonprofit hospital system in the United States had its beginning in Philadelphia in 1751 with the founding of the Pennsylvania Hospital. Still in operation, this institution is the oldest community hospital in the nation. In addition, it can lay claim to being the oldest of all United States hospitals because it was the first institution in this country incorporated solely for the purpose of providing care to the physically and mentally ill regardless of economic status, race, or religion, although several almshouses with infirmary facilities were founded earlier and later evolved into hospitals.

The Pennsylvania Hospital had its origin in the desire of a Philadelphia physician, Dr. Thomas Bond, to have a facility in which he could practice surgery and treat patients. After failing to sufficiently interest his friends and colleagues in a hospital project, Dr. Bond enlisted the aid and support of Benjamin Franklin. The latter subscribed generously to the project himself, publicized the need for such an institution, and solicited contributions from influential citizens. In addition, Franklin was successful in obtaining a grant of two thousand pounds from the Provincial Assembly of Pennsylvania for the construction of the hospital on the condition that a similar sum be raised through public subscription. Pennsylvania Hospital opened its doors to patients in 1755, and Benjamin Franklin served as the hospital's first clerk and as president from 1755 to 1757.

Other early community hospitals include the New York Hospital, established in New York City in 1771; the Massachusetts General Hospital, founded in 1811 in Boston; McLean Hospital, a psychiatric institution established in Waverly, Massachusetts, in 1811; and the New Haven Hospital, incorporated in 1826 in New Haven, Connecticut.

Measures of Significance. Completely accurate statistics on community hospitals are not available and it must be recognized that the following figures are nothing more than rough estimates based on the limited information that could be obtained.

In 1956 there were more than 2000 community hospitals in the United States. They had a combined capacity of approximately 230,000 beds and, during the year, admitted nearly 7,400,000 patients, or about 33 admissions per bed. The average daily census in the same period was around 170,000 patients and the average occupancy rate was roughly 74 per cent.

Most of the community hospitals are short-term, general-acute institutions; only a small percentage provide care of a specialized nature. Typically, they are medium in size with an average capacity slightly in excess of 100 beds.

An estimated 342,000 persons were employed in community hospitals in 1956, or more than two employees per patient.

These institutions are well distributed throughout the country, and most states have a relatively large number of community hospitals.

Financial Data. The total expenditures of community hospitals in 1956 were estimated to exceed $1.4 billion, or more than $23.00 per patient day. Payroll expenses were around $880 million, and the payroll component of total expenses was over 60 per cent. In the same year, total assets were estimated at $3.16 billion, or roughly $14,000 per bed.

Community hospitals serve a paying clientele, and operating income is derived almost entirely from patient revenue. Capital funds for construction and expansion come from operating reserves, endowments, community campaigns, Hill-Burton grants from the federal government, and loans from banks, insurance companies, and other commercial sources.

Educational Activities. Very little information is available on the educational and research activities of community hospitals. Certainly many of these institutions operate approved professional nursing schools, and a smaller — but nevertheless significant — number have approved programs for practical nurses. It is also believed that a high percentage of the larger community hospitals, particularly those in metropolitan areas, are approved for residencies and internships by the American Medical Association.

Administration. Most community hospitals are administered by persons outside of the medical profession. The administrator is selected by the trustees or directors of the hospital and is directly responsible to them for the management of the institution.

Medical Staff. The medical staff in the majority of community hospitals is organized in a manner similar to that illustrated earlier in the chapter by the Uniontown Hospital and the Charles T. Miller Hospital. Size permitting, the staff is divided into major clinical services. Each service is headed by a chief who is usually elected by the service itself but, in some cases, is appointed by the governing board of the hospital.

The staff elects, generally on an annual basis, one of its members to serve as the president or chief of the staff. He coordinates his functions with the hospital administrator and directs the staff activities.

A joint conference committee, normally composed of an equal number of staff members and trustees or directors, is frequently maintained in community hospitals to solve problems of both a medical and an administrative nature.

Trends. Community hospitals have increased significantly, both in number and in size, in the past decade. However, future trends for these institutions are difficult to determine and are apparently dependent on the future of the voluntary hospital system in this country. Hospital costs have risen enormously in recent years. Though this increase in costs is justifiable, the American public has become alarmed. If costs continue to rise as is expected, it is questionable how much longer our citizens will be willing to assume the responsibility of financing hospital and medical care for themselves. If they choose to preserve the voluntary hospital system, community hospitals will continue to grow and expand, though less rapidly than they have in the past few years. However, if the public chooses some sort of governmental support or control, both the voluntary system and community hospitals will suffer accordingly.

JEWISH HOSPITALS

Jewish-sponsored hospitals in the United States are similar, in at least one respect, to hospitals operated under Protestant and Catholic auspices — they are sectarian hospitals with a nonsectarian intake or admission policy. However, they differ from Catholic and Protestant hospitals in that they are not owned or operated by or related to any religious institutions. They are the product of the Jewish community rather than of one or several Jewish temples or synagogues.

Organizational Structure and Governing Authority. Jewish hospitals follow the pattern under which the "community" and most other voluntary, nonprofit hospitals are organized. In all cases, as far as is known, ownership and operating control are vested in a board of trustees which is completely secular in character. Membership on these governing boards is usually open to persons of all races and/or religions. In actual practice, however, the boards are frequently composed entirely of Jewish individuals.

History of Growth and Development. In 1654 the first group of Jewish immigrants arrived in the United States and settled in New Amsterdam, a colony of Holland. Under what became known as the Toleration Act, these Jewish immigrants had to guarantee to Holland, through Peter Stuyvesant, the colony's governor, that they would take care of their own, the sick as well as the poor. Although these terms are, of course, no longer binding, the Jewish community in America still continues to provide social and health services for a large share of its people.

Perhaps the first Jewish hospital in this country was Jews Hospital, now known as Mt. Sinai, established in New York City in 1852. Other Jewish hospitals were founded at approximately the same time in Philadelphia, Baltimore, Cincinnati, New Orleans, San Francisco, and Chicago.

Another large group of Jewish hospitals opened their doors in the decade from 1900 to 1910 as a result of the heavy wave of Jewish immigrants to the United States at the turn of the century. Jewish hospitals also experienced accelerated growth in the periods following the two World Wars. By 1956, every city having a Jewish community of more than 30,000, with the exception of Washington, D.C., had at least one hospital and there were hospitals in ten cities with a Jewish population of less than 30,000.

When Jewish hospitals were first established in this country, they were intended to be used exclusively by Jewish people. Approximately ten to twenty years later, this sectarian admission policy was altered and both Jews and non-Jews were accepted as patients. Once altered, this admission policy has never been changed and today over 50 per cent of the patients in Jewish hospitals are non-Jews. On the other hand, it is estimated that more than one half of the Jewish people needing hospitalization in the United States are cared for in non-Jewish institutions.

The following are the principal reasons for the establishment of Jewish hospitals in this country:

1. The concentration of large Jewish populations in various cities and metropolitan areas and the desire of the Jewish people to care for their own.

2. The desire of the Jewish population to do its share in providing better hospital care for people of all faiths and to contribute to the advancement of medical knowledge through research.

3. The desire to provide a Jewish environment where Jewish patients could adhere to their traditional dietary laws and religious customs.

4. The necessity of providing institutions for Jewish physicians to admit patients because of the restrictions against such doctors in many non-Jewish hospitals.

5. The necessity of providing institutions where Jewish medical school graduates could receive internship and residency training because of the discrimination practiced against such graduates in some of the non-Jewish teaching hospitals.

Of the above, the last two reasons have diminished considerably in significance since the end of World War II.

Measures of Significance. There were sixty-eight known Jewish hospitals in the United States and Canada in 1956. Sixty-three of these institutions reported statistics for that year to the Council of Jewish Federations and Welfare Funds. The following information pertains only to the fifty-nine reporting hospitals located in this country.

Among these fifty-nine institutions were forty-one general, two psychiatric, eight tuberculosis, six chronic and convalescent, and two "other" hospitals. Their combined capacity was 15,582 beds and 1864 bassinets. During the year, they admitted nearly 427,000 patients, or more than 27 admissions per bed. Over 13,000 patients were in these hospitals on any given day and the average occupancy rate exceeded 83 per cent.

More than 32,000 persons were employed in these hospitals, or roughly 2.5 employees per patient.

In general, Jewish hospitals are quite large. Nearly 60 per cent of the reporting hospitals had over 200 beds in 1956 and the average capacity was approximately 260 beds. Their large size is undoubtedly due to their location in or near metropolitan centers which have a substantial Jewish population.

Although each of the American Hospital Association's nine geographic regions contained at least one of the reporting Jewish hospitals, nearly 70 per cent of the institutions were located east of the Mississippi River. The heaviest concentration was in the Middle Atlantic region, and New York City alone had seventeen Jewish hospitals, or approximately 28 per cent of the total.

About 59 per cent of the reporting Jewish hospitals were accredited by the Joint Commission on Accreditation of Hospitals. In addition, 94 per cent were members of the American Hospital Association and 91 per cent belonged to state and/or regional associations.

Financial Data. The fifty-nine reporting Jewish hospitals expended an estimated $140 million in 1956 and the expense per patient day was approximately $29.00. Estimated payroll expenses exceeded $90 million and the payroll component of the total expenditures was nearly 64 per cent, slightly less than the national average of 65.6 per cent for all hospitals.

In that year, approximately 74 per cent of the hospitals' operating income was derived from patients and third parties for services rendered, 7 per cent from public funds, 6.5 per cent from local Jewish federations and welfare funds, 6 per cent from contributions, 2 per cent from various Community Chests, and 4.5 per cent from other sources.

Total assets of the fifty-nine hospitals exceeded $300 million in 1956, or more than $19,000 per bed. There is a strong tendency in Jewish hospitals to construct and expand with funds raised for that specific purpose rather than borrow the necessary money. Consequently, campaigns conducted by the various hospitals and/or local Jewish welfare federations are the major source of capital funds.

Educational and Research Activities. Jewish hospitals in the United States are extremely active in education and research. Undoubtedly, the high degree of participation in these fields is partly due to the fact that most Jewish hospitals are of sufficient size to support such activities and the metropolitan centers in which many of these institutions are located are a good source of teaching patients. However, the extent to which Jewish hospitals and their governing organizations maintain and support education and research is also indicative of the great value they place upon such programs.

Over 70 per cent of the reporting Jewish hospitals were approved for residencies by the American Medical Association in 1956, approximately 60 per cent had internship approval and nearly 25 per cent were reportedly affiliated with medical schools. In addition, around 30 per cent of the hospitals and state-approved professional nursing schools and approximately 5 per cent operated approved practical nursing programs.

In 1953 research was being conducted in at least thirteen Jewish hospitals either as an integral part of the hospital program or as a separate research service. During that year, the total research budget in these institutions was over 2.5 million dollars. Research programs in Jewish hospitals are financially supported in several ways: by grants from foundations and the federal government, by research funds from local Jewish welfare federations, by separate research corporations, and by funds received from women's auxiliaries.

Administration. In general, Jewish hospitals are administratively similar to other voluntary, nonprofit hospitals. However, Jewish hospitals have a relatively higher proportion of administrators who are members of the medical profession than do other voluntary patterns.

Medical Staff. The organization of the medical staffs in Jewish hospitals is also similar to the pattern followed in other voluntary, nonprofit institutions. Staff membership is limited to qualified, licensed physicians but there are no restrictions on the basis of race, color, or creed.

In recent years a number of Jewish hospitals have employed full-time chiefs of major clinical services who are responsible for services, beds, teaching, and research.

Council of Jewish Federations and Welfare Funds, Incorporated. There is no formal association of Jewish hospitals. However, all hospitals are associated with local community planning bodies such as Jewish welfare federations or community councils. Through these federations and councils the hospitals may be indirectly associated with a national planning body called the Council of Jewish Federations and Welfare Funds, Incorporated.

This Council was established in 1932 as the outgrowth of lay and professional experience in three earlier national organizations. It is a membership association of more than two hundred local Jewish federations, welfare funds, and community councils in the United States and Canada and was established and is governed and maintained by these groups. The constitution declared the Council's objectives were "to offer a medium for the consideration of common interests and problems," and within the framework of the constitution, the Council set the following basic goals for itself: (1) to develop and promote standards and principles of effective community organizations; (2) to foster cooperation on an inter-city basis among Jewish communities; (3) to facilitate the relationship of local communities to national and overseas organizations.

Most of the Jewish service agencies provide the Council with annual statistics on services rendered, income, expenditures, etc., and the Council publishes an analysis of these statistics in a yearbook, in a manner somewhat similar to that in which the data for all hospitals are compiled and published annually by the American Hospital Association.

Trends. As stated previously, some of the reasons for originally establishing Jewish hospitals are diminishing in importance. Consequently, while Jewish hospitals will probably experience a gradual growth in the future, it appears that growth will be considerably less rapid than it has been in the past.

INDUSTRIAL HOSPITALS

Located throughout the United States, particularly in the West, are a number of hospitals which are classified as "industrial" because of their association with certain industries or business enterprises. These hospitals are usually operated as part of a health plan providing medical and hospital care to employees and, in many cases, their dependents.

Organizational Structure and Governing Authority. Industrial health plans vary a great deal in their organizational structure and governing authority. In 1949 the Social Security Administration of the federal government reported on 149 industrial health plans, approximately one fourth of the estimated number of such plans in the United States. Thirty of these plans were sponsored by employers, fifty-nine by employees, forty-four by both employers and employees, fourteen by unions, and two by employers and unions.

In many of the plans sponsored wholly or partly by employees, the actual operating organization is an employee beneficial association. Many of these associations are completely free and independent of both employers and unions. However, about one half of the companies initiating or encouraging such associations exercise some degree of control and supervision over association affairs.

Membership in the various industrial health plans is usually voluntary, although a few companies make it a condition of employment. Most of the plans operate on a service basis, as opposed to a cash indemnity basis, and usually provide comprehensive medical and hospital care.

Approximately 59 per cent of the known industrial hospitals in 1956 were associated with railroads and the remaining 41 per cent were connected with other enterprises such as tire, mining, sulphur, oil, and copper companies.

The employee beneficial association of the Northern Pacific Railroad operates one of the best-known industrial health plans. The following discussion of the organizational structure of this association is presented to provide a better understanding of the industrial pattern of hospital ownership and control.

The Northern Pacific Beneficial Association. In continuous operation since 1882, this employee-employer-sponsored association serves any point on the Northern Pacific Railway lines. Its membership consists of the employees of the Northern Pacific Railway Company, employees of the Northern Pacific Beneficial Association, employees of corporations in which the Northern Pacific owns 50 per cent or more of the stock, and a limited number of employees of the Railway Express

Agency. Dependents are not eligible for membership and are not entitled to association benefits.

Hospitalization is provided in four hospitals — two in Montana, and one each in Minnesota and Washington — owned and operated by a separate but interrelated corporation, the Northern Pacific Beneficial Association Hospitals, Inc. In emergencies, treatment may also be given in other hospitals.

The association employs, on a full- or part-time basis, approximately four hundred physicians located at various points along the Northern Pacific lines. They staff the hospitals and furnish medical services in their private offices or in the homes of association members throughout the system.

Although separate entities, both the beneficial association and the hospital corporation are governed by the same board of directors and executive committee. The board is composed of twenty-four directors — fifteen elected by the association members from within the membership and eight appointed by the chief operating officer of the railroad, preferably from heads of departments. The chief operating officer serves as an ex officio member of the board.

The executive committee consists of four directors, elected by the board, and the president of the Northern Pacific Beneficial Association, who serves as an ex officio member of the committee. The president is the executive officer of the association. He is elected by the board of directors for a four-year term and reports to the board annually or to the executive committee when it meets.

History of Growth and Development. The industrial plans were among the first health insurance plans developed in the United States. Many were established as far back as 1860 and 1870. The primary purpose of these early plans was to pay cash benefits to employees when they were sick; medical care provisions were rarely included.

Apparently the first industrial hospital was the Southern Pacific General, founded in 1869 in Sacramento, California. This institution — now located in San Francisco — is not only still in operation but is currently the largest hospital of its kind. Most of the other hospitals were added in the period from 1870 to 1890 and in the early 1900s. A few industrial hospitals established themselves just prior to World War II and another small number were started in the postwar period.

The various industrial health plans and industrial hospitals were established for a number of different reasons. Many of the older plans and hospitals were developed for employees of hazardous occupations — mining, lumbering, railroading, etc. — who were working in remote areas with no medical facilities. Other plans resulted from Workmen's Compensation legislation in the early 1900s, which made the employer responsible for providing medical care to injured employees. Some of the industrial health plans were developed by various concerns as part of a welfare program to win employee loyalty and discourage union organization. During World War II, wages were stabilized and a number of industries established health plans as one of many fringe benefits designed to attract and maintain employees. Still other plans resulted from collective bargaining agreements between unions and employers. Finally, many industrial and business enterprises have found it economical to support or contribute to health plans because, in safeguarding the employees' health, such plans have reduced absenteeism, made production more profitable, and improved relations between labor and management.

Measures of Significance. Industrial medicine has a greater effect on the nation's health than that represented by the statistics on industrial hospitals. Many industrial health plans provide both medical and hospital care. However, most plans use existing community facilities and only a few operate their own hospitals.

Completely accurate statistics on industrial hospitals are difficult to obtain. The following information pertains to the fifty-four hospitals which were known to be associated with various industrial and business enterprises in 1956.

The combined capacity of the fifty-four hospitals was 4583 beds—approximately one per cent of the total nongovernmental, nonprofit hospital beds in the United States. During 1956 these industrial institutions admitted 110,033 patients, or slightly more than 24 admissions per bed. The average daily census was 2889 patients and the occupancy rate exceeded 63 per cent.

A total of 4451 persons were employed in the fifty-four hospitals, or more than 1.5 employees per patient.

The hospitals ranged in size from the 13-bed San Juan Miners Hospital in Ouray, Colorado, to the 450-bed Southern Pacific General in San Francisco. Twenty-five hospitals, or 46 per cent of the total, had less than 50 beds; 74 per cent had fewer than 100 beds. Only four hospitals, or less than 7.5 per cent of the total, had more than 200 beds.

With the exception of New England, all of the American Hospital Association's geographic regions had one or more industrial hospitals. However, thirty-eight hospitals — or approximately 70 per cent — were located west of the Mississippi River. The mountain region, which had fewer hospitals of *all* types than any of the other geographic areas, contained the greatest proportion — nearly 28 per cent — of the industrial institutions.

All but one of the hospitals provided short-term, general-acute care. The one exception was a long-term, tuberculosis institution.

Patterns of Hospital Ownership and Control

Nearly 56 per cent of these industrial hospitals were accredited by the Joint Commission on Accreditation of Hospitals in 1956. Forty-six per cent were members of the American Hospital Association and over 57 per cent belonged to state and/or regional hospital associations.

Financial Data. An estimated $23 million was expended in 1956 in operating the fifty-four hospitals, and the expenses per patient day approximated $21.80.

The payroll expenses exceeded $12.5 million. The payroll component of total expenses was more than 55 per cent as compared with the national average of 61 per cent for all nonprofit, short-term hospitals.

The operating income of industrial hospitals comes primarily from dues paid in advance by the employees, from regular contributions by the employers, or both. Additional revenue is received in some of these institutions from patients who are not employees of the industrial concern involved or who are not members of the employee association operating the hospital.

The total capitalization of the industrial hospitals in the United States in 1956 exceeded $18 million, or approximately $4000 per bed. This figure is extremely low in comparison with other hospital patterns. However, it must be remembered that most industrial hospitals were built many years ago, when construction costs were low and when hospitals did not find it necessary to provide as many services and as many different types of accommodation as they do today.

Capital funds for new construction and expansion come from operating surpluses; from contributions and donations by employees, employee associations, unions, and industrial concerns; and from loans obtained from industry and commercial banking sources.

Educational Activities. Industrial hospitals carry on proportionately fewer educational activities than most of the other hospital patterns. Undoubtedly, this is partly due to their relatively small size and the consequent lack of the patients, staff, and facilities necessary to support such programs.

Seven hospitals, or less than 13 per cent of the total, had been approved for residencies by the American Medical Association in 1956. Four hospitals were approved for internships and only one maintained an affiliation with a medical school. Also, only one hospital operated an approved professional nursing program.

Administration. The role assumed by the person occupying the top administrative position in an industrial hospital varies with the type of industry with which the hospital is associated. In several hospitals the chief executive is a physician who serves in a dual capacity as both administrator and medical director. The administration of other industrial hospitals is in the hands of a nonmedical administrator who coordinates his functions with a medical director or chief of staff.

Medical Staff. The medical staffs in the larger industrial hospitals are organized by clinical services under the direction of a medical director or chief of staff. However, the staffs in most of the industrial hospitals have too small a membership to be organized in such a manner.

Many industrial hospitals are staffed wholly or in part by physicians who are either full- or part-time employees of the organization controlling the institution.

Trends. In recent years there has been a significant increase in the number of industrial health plans. As stated previously, many are developing as the result of collective bargaining agreements, and industry is finding such plans economical. Consequently, it would seem reasonable to expect that the number of industrial plans will continue to increase in the future.

On the other hand, the number of industrial hospitals and beds should remain relatively constant and may even decline. There are two reasons for this seeming contradiction. First of all, industry is no longer expanding into remote, isolated areas with no medical facilities. Such areas have virtually ceased to exist in the United States and adequate hospitals are present in almost every section of the country. As a result, it is no longer necessary for industry to build its own institutions. Secondly, hospitals of this type are finding it increasingly difficult to break even financially as they are generally quite small and usually have a low occupancy rate. Consequently, from an economical standpoint, it would appear to be unwise to construct more industrial hospitals if existing community facilities are available and adequate.

COOPERATIVE HOSPITALS

Cooperative hospitals and cooperative health plans represent one of the most direct attempts now being made by groups of American people to solve the problem of medical economics by their own efforts.

Health cooperatives are formal associations organized and controlled by the users or purchasers of health services. Although they vary tremendously in their organizational structure and in the services and benefits they provide, most cooperative health plans (1) provide comprehensive health care of both a preventive and curative nature; (2) require prepayment by members to budget the costs of medical care; (3) provide for democratic control by the members; (4) utilize group medical practice; (5) provide assurance that there will be no interference by laymen with the practice of medicine.

Organizational Structure and Governing Authority. Most cooperative health associations are incorporated. In some states they are or-

131

ganized under "cooperative" statutes while in others they are established under "nonprofit association" laws.

In some states, only physicians may incorporate nonprofit medical service plans. A health cooperative in such a state is forced to set up two parallel associations: (1) an *incorporated association*, which owns the hospital and clinic facilities and which permits tax-exempt operations, and (2) an *unincorporated association*, which contracts with and compensates the physicians associated with the health plan and receives premium payments from the members of the plan.

The governing boards of almost all cooperative health associations are elected by the members in annual meetings provided for in the by-laws of the associations. The boards usually meet once a month and are composed of from five to eleven directors who serve for terms of one to four years. Most associations require the directors to be members of the association. The governing board of a cooperative health association is directly responsible to the membership for the operation of the association and, in most cases, for any facilities which the association may own. A manager is usually selected by the board to administer the affairs of the association. If the association owns or operates a hospital and/or clinic, he may also be responsible for these facilities.

Characteristics of Cooperative Health Plans. Cooperative health plans vary enormously in the services and benefits they afford their members. Some are direct service plans operating hospitals and/or clinics while others are indemnity plans with no facilities of their own. Some are comprehensive plans affording both hospital and medical care benefits while others are more restrictive in the services they provide. Employers participate in a few plans by paying all or a portion of their employees' premiums and dues. One characteristic common to the direct service plans is the encouragement of disease prevention and health maintenance as well as the cure of disease.

History of Growth and Development. Cooperatives are not a new development in this country. For many years, groups of American people — particularly those residing in rural areas — have organized cooperatives to operate creameries, mills, and a number of other enterprises. However, only in recent years have cooperative associations been utilized to any great extent to solve health and medical economic problems.

Immigrants were the originators of cooperative medicine in the United States. La Société Française de Bienfaisance Mutuelle de San Francisco, a benevolent society composed of French immigrants, established a mutual-aid hospital in San Francisco, California, in 1851. Although apparently no longer a cooperative institution, it is still in operation and is presently known as the French Hospital.

During the 1890s, Spanish and Cuban immigrants settled in and around Tampa, Florida. Strangers to America, they banded together in "centros" which served as the core of their social and cultural life. Democratically controlled organizations operating in a cooperative manner, these "centros" also provided the immigrants with a wide variety of welfare benefits, including medical and hospital care. Shortly after the turn of the century, two of them — the Centro Espanol and the Centro Asturiano — acquired their own hospitals, still in operation today.

Probably the first health plan to employ all the principles of cooperative medicine was founded in Elk City, Oklahoma, in 1929. Pioneered by the father of the cooperative health movement in the United States, Dr. Michael A. Shadid, this plan was established with no capital and a membership of twelve families. In 1956 the plan was operating a combination hospital-clinic of 75 beds which served approximately 7000 beneficiaries and an equal number of nonmember patients.

Cooperative health associations experienced their greatest growth following World War II. At present, there are nearly one hundred such associations serving an estimated two million persons. Most of these health cooperatives are in rural areas; however, a significant number have been established in urban centers in the past few years.

All types of health insurance plan which involve the group practice of medicine have encountered opposition from the medical profession on both a national and local level. This is particularly true of cooperative health plans. Organized medicine has exerted pressure on state legislatures to restrict or prevent the formation of such plans, and physicians who are associated with health cooperatives have been professionally ostracized. Although cooperative health plans are still being opposed by the medical profession in some areas of the country, the situation has improved tremendously in recent years because of less forceful opposition.

Measures of Significance. Accurate statistics pertaining to cooperative hospitals are not available and it must be recognized that the following figures are nothing more than rough estimates.

In 1956 from thirty to forty of the nearly one hundred cooperative health plans operated a hospital, usually in combination with a clinic or health center. Total capacity of these hospitals was around 1000 beds, and about 30,000 patients were admitted during the year. The cooperative hospitals for which figures were available had an occupancy rate of less than 50 per cent; consequently the average daily census in all cooperative institutions was estimated to be under 500 patients.

All of the known cooperative hospitals were short-term, general-acute institutions. They were typically quite small, the largest one having only 81 beds, and their average capacity was less than 39 beds.

More than 1000 persons were estimated to be employed in cooperative hospitals in 1956, or just over two employees per patient.

Approximately 95 per cent of the known cooperative hospitals were members of state and/or regional hospital associations; more than 75 per cent belonged to the national organization. Less than 15 per cent had been accredited by the Joint Commission on Accreditation of Hospitals.

Over 80 per cent of the known cooperative hospitals were located west of the Mississippi River and more than 50 per cent were in the American Hospital Association's West South Central region.

Most of the cooperative health plans were established by people living in sparsely populated rural areas; only a few of the hospitals and plans are located in urban centers. The distribution of cooperative hospitals and health plans is also affected by the statutes in the various states regulating the formation and operation of health cooperatives.

Financial Data. The operating expenses of cooperative hospitals were estimated at more than $5 million in 1956, or from $20 to $25 per patient day. The payroll component of total expenses was over 53 per cent. Total capital invested in cooperative hospitals was estimated at six million dollars, or more than $6000 per bed.

The principal sources of operating income are the prepaid premiums and dues received from health plan members. Income is also received from hospital patients who are not members of the cooperative associations.

Capital funds come from operating reserves, community campaigns, grants from the federal government, and loans from banks and other commercial sources.

Most of the cooperative health plans are financially solvent, although many of the direct service plans carry an indebtedness due to the acquisition and construction of physical facilities. A few cooperative plans have had, and are having, a difficult time financially because they were not established on a sound actuarial basis. Poor selection of risks, small memberships, heavy turnover, and premium rates that were set too low have taken, and are taking, their toll.

Educational Activities. None of the known cooperative hospitals were approved by the American Medical Association for internships and residencies in 1956, none were affiliated with a medical school, and none operated an approved professional nursing school. An approved practical nursing school was in operation at the Community Hospital in Elk City, Oklahoma.

Administration. As previously indicated, the governing board of a cooperative health plan usually hires an individual to manage the affairs of the association. If the plan operates its own clinic and/or hospital, the manager of the association is often given the additional responsibility of administering these facilities.

Medical Staff. Cooperative hospitals and health centers are usually staffed by groups of physicians who contract with the various health plans for the services they render. They are compensated in a number of different ways: salary, fee for service, fee per patient, or combinations of these and other payment methods.

Physicians who are associated with a cooperative hospital and health plan must have at least the same qualifications as those required of private practitioners and, to avoid the possibility of lay interference in the practice of medicine, these physicians are, in all cases, selected for the cooperative association by other members of the medical profession. Nevertheless, in some areas of the United States, physicians who are associated with cooperative plans have been accused of engaging in the "corporate practice of medicine" and have been barred from local medical societies and other professional organizations. In some instances the opposition of organized medicine has had such a strangulating effect on the activities of the cooperative associations that they have found it necessary to bring suit against the medical societies under the antitrust laws of the state and federal governments and have won several cases.

Group Health Federation of America. The Group Health Federation of America (formerly known as the Cooperative Health Federation of America) was organized in 1946 at Two Harbors, Minnesota, by nine charter health plan members. Today it is recognized as the voice and spokesman for democratically controlled cooperative and prepayment group health plans. In 1958 it consisted of twenty-four regular members, including the largest and best-known cooperative and group health plans: Group Health Association, Inc., of Washington, D.C., Group Health Cooperative of Puget Sound, and Health Insurance Plan of Greater New York. The federation also had more than one hundred associate members. Among these were many of the major regional cooperatives, labor unions, and farmers' organizations.

The federation carries on a number of activities to assist and guide the development of cooperative and group health plans. It provides a legal and legislative service, arranges for consultants, and helps to secure personnel. It also serves as a central source of information on medical economic problems and provides for the exchange of such information among its members by conducting annual institutes and by publishing and distributing newsletters and bulletins.

Trends. There are several factors limiting the potential growth of cooperative hospitals and cooperative health associations:

1. The statutes in force in some states restrict or prevent the establishment of such associations by laymen.

2. The rural location of many cooperative health plans and/or the opposition of the medical profession in some areas make it difficult to attract professional personnel.

3. In some sections of the country, the poorer population groups have such a meager income that they are unable to participate in cooperative health plans even though the costs are prepaid and the premiums are low.

However, despite these limiting factors, cooperative hospitals and health associations experienced a phenomenal growth in the five-year period following World War II. Since 1950 they have developed at a steady but less rapid pace, and it is reasonable to expect this gradual growth to continue in the future.

Cooperative health plans will undoubtedly continue to use existing hospitals and clinics wherever possible. When such facilities are not present, health cooperatives will be forced to construct or acquire their own. Consequently, it appears there will be a small but relatively insignificant increase in the number of cooperative hospitals in the coming years.

THE MINERS MEMORIAL HOSPITAL ASSOCIATION

"A hospital chain 250 miles long" aptly describes the ten hospitals which were built and are administered by the Miners Memorial Hospital Association, a nonprofit corporation established and financed by the United Mine Workers of America Welfare and Retirement Fund (see Fig. 20).

The hospitals are located in Kentucky, Virginia, and West Virginia, in an area 250 miles long and 100 miles wide. Almost one third of the nation's coal tonnage is produced in this region and one third of the members of the United Mine Workers of America (UMWA) reside in the area. The ten hospitals — three base or central hospitals and seven smaller, affiliated hospitals — serve a population of approximately three hundred thousand miners and one million dependents.

Organizational Structure and Governing Authority. The UMWA Welfare and Retirement Fund is a charitable trust, established in 1946 as a result of wage negotiations between coal operators and the UMWA. However, the fund is a separate entity, independent of both the union and the operators. Its purpose is to provide, out of royalty revenues from the production of coal, benefits to UMWA members and their families and dependents, including hospital and medical care.

The board of trustees of the fund consists of three members: one

Figure 20. The United Mine Workers of America Welfare
and Retirement Fund, 1956

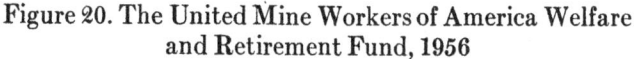

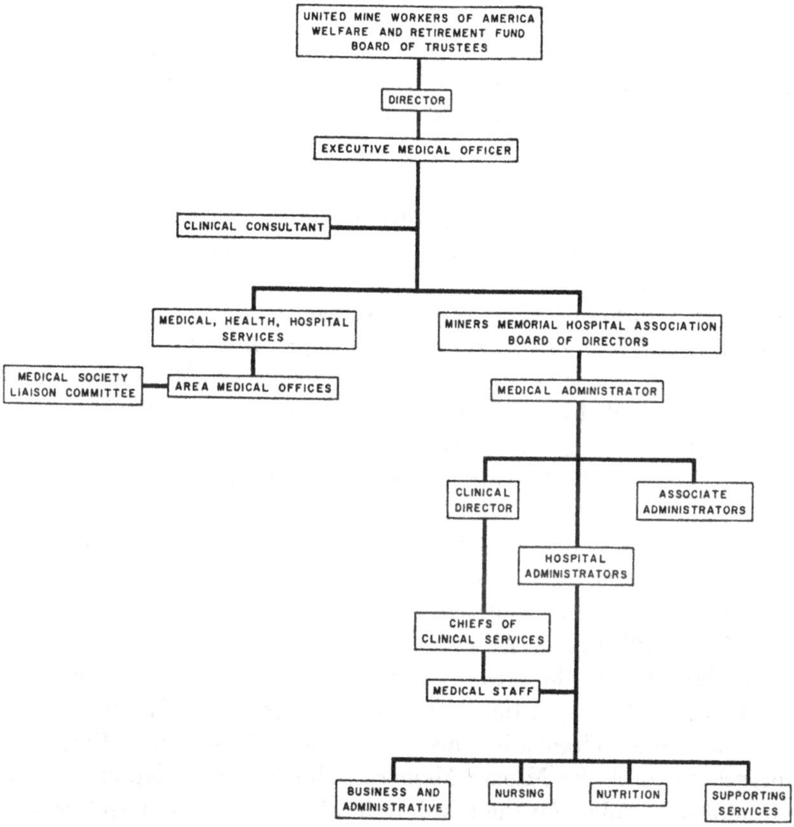

representing the union, one representing the bituminous coal industry,
and one neutral member appointed by the other two. As of this writing, the chairman and chief executive officer of the fund is John L.
Lewis, president of the UMWA. The director of the fund is the neutral
trustee.

The directors of the Miners Memorial Hospital Association are all
fund employees and the association's president is an assistant of the
executive medical officer of the fund. The medical administrator is a
physician who is responsible for the over-all medical and administrative
management of the association.

The ten hospitals are highly coordinated. The three base or central
hospitals at Harlan and South Williamson, Kentucky, and Beckley,
West Virginia, are located in natural trade centers. The Harlan hospital
has four smaller community hospitals affiliated with it. The Williamson

hospital is affiliated with three community hospitals. Because of its geographical location, the central hospital at Beckley operates as a single unit. The community hospitals generally handle the more routine medical and surgical cases on both an inpatient and outpatient basis. Patients requiring specialized care are usually referred to the central hospitals, although specialists also travel to the community hospitals for some of the complicated cases.

All services directly touching on patient care, such as medical records, are present in each of the hospitals. However, purchasing, payroll accounting, supervisory training, menu planning, and maintenance are centralized. The efficiency generated by this coordinated and centralized system has reduced operating costs considerably.

History of Growth and Development. In providing hospital and medical care to its beneficiaries, the UMWA Welfare and Retirement Fund originally intended to supplement, not supplant, existing facilities. Although some areas served by the fund were sadly lacking the resources to provide proper health care, the fund hoped that the security of sure-payment for services rendered beneficiaries would spur new construction and raise the quality of patient care. However, in 1951, the fund's Medical Advisory Committee reported that a dearth of adequate medical facilities persisted and that some hospitals were so bad the fund would not utilize them. As a result, it was decided to build a network of ten hospitals in the area needing them most. In October 1951, the fund approved loans to three nonprofit corporations in Kentucky, Virginia, and West Virginia for this construction. These corporations were merged to form the Miners Memorial Hospital Association in 1955. Ground was broken for the first hospital in 1953 and all hospitals were in operation at the time of the dedication on June 2, 1956.

In principle, the ten hospitals operate much like any other nongovernmental, nonprofit hospital. They are open to all patients, although beneficiaries of the UMWA Welfare and Retirement Fund have a priority for beds in case of a shortage. As UMWA members are located in all parts of the United States, the fund also uses other hospitals for the care of its beneficiaries.

Measures of Significance. All ten hospitals are general-acute institutions. During 1957 their combined capacity was 1023 beds and they admitted over 27,000 patients, or about 26 admissions per bed. The average daily census was 672 patients and the average occupancy rate was around 66 per cent.

In the same period, the average capacity of the hospitals was just over 102 beds and they ranged in size from the 50-bed institution at Pikeville, Kentucky, to the 193-bed Beckley Memorial Hospital in

Beckley, West Virginia. Each hospital is designed so that its bed complement can be doubled without rearranging service facilities.

All ten hospitals were accredited by the Joint Commission on Accreditation of Hospitals in 1957 and were members of the American Hospital Association and state and regional hospital associations.

More than 2050 persons were employed in the hospitals in 1957, or approximately three employees per patient. Wherever possible, the hospitals are employing disabled miners and their families or the families of miners who were killed on the job. It is conservatively estimated that about 240 employees currently fall into this category, of which around ninety are disabled miners who have received training for hospital positions in state and federal vocational rehabilitation programs.

The senior personnel in the various professional and technical services in the central hospitals have the over-all responsibility for these services in the affiliated community hospitals. Such senior personnel coordinate their activities with the administrators of the affiliated hospitals to avoid encroaching on the administrators' responsibility and authority. Thus, for example, the smaller institutions can get along reasonably well without a professional dietitian on their staffs.

Financial Data. The UMWA Welfare and Retirement fund receives a royalty of forty cents a ton on all coal produced by the operators signing the National Bituminous Coal Wage Agreement. In the 1955 fiscal year, the fund received over $129 million in royalties and expended $119 million.

During that year, 1,605,486 days of hospital care were provided to over 95,000 beneficiaries in 1599 hospitals in forty-five states, the District of Columbia, and Alaska. The total cost of the medical and hospital program exceeded $42 million, or approximately 35 per cent of the fund's total expenditures.

In 1957 the ten hospitals operated by the Miners Memorial Hospital Association expended more than $13 million. Payroll expenses were nearly $8.5 million, or over 61 per cent of the total. These institutions receive per diem rates from the fund for care rendered to fund beneficiaries. The hospitals also obtain some operating income from other patients who are not beneficiaries of the fund.

The total capital invested in the ten hospitals was estimated to exceed $25 million in 1957, or about $24,500 per bed. All money for the construction of the hospitals was obtained from the UMWA Welfare and Retirement Fund through loans which are meticulously secured by first deeds of trust on all property and buildings acquired by the hospital association.

Educational Activities. None of the hospitals had intern or residency programs in 1957, nor were any affiliated with medical schools. However, the teaching and training of physicians and other personnel is an integral part of the Miners Memorial Hospital Association program and it is anticipated that both internships and residencies will be offered as soon as hospital operations have stabilized and there has been an opportunity to gauge the educational potential of the various medical specialties. In addition, the association eventually expects to affiliate with several medical schools. An active program of postgraduate education is also contemplated for members of the various medical staffs.

The hospital at Harlan, Kentucky, is currently affiliated with a professional nursing school, and the hospital at South Williamson, Kentucky, is operating an approved school for practical nurses. The association also has coordinated training programs for supervisors, nurse aides, technologists, and other personnel.

Administration. The association maintains a central office in Washington, D.C., and a field office in Williamson, West Virginia. The staff at the Washington office includes the medical administrator, clinical director, associate clinical director, and the associate administrators for business services and special services. The field office staff includes the associate administrators for personnel services, nursing services and education, and property services. The associate administrators are specialists in their particular areas and act as "circuit riding" advisors to the individual hospital administrators.

Community hospital administrators are responsible to the administrators of the central hospitals with which they are affiliated. The three central hospital administrators are, in turn, responsible to the medical administrator of the association. An administrative committee, made up of all ten hospital administrators and the medical administrator and members of his staff, meets regularly to formulate organizational and management policies.

Medical Staff. The medical functions of each hospital are organized into the basic divisions of medicine, surgery, obstetrics, pediatrics, clinical pathology and radiology, and such other services as may be determined by the clinical director with the approval of the medical administrator.

The chief of clinical services of each hospital is appointed by the association's board of directors and is responsible for coordinating medical services, clinical investigation, and teaching. He serves as a liaison between the medical staff and the hospital administrator in medical matters and collaborates with the administrator in matters of mutual concern. He is an ex officio member of all medical staff and hospital administration committees. The chiefs of clinical services in the community hospitals are responsible to the chiefs of clinical services in the central hospitals with which they are affiliated. They, in turn, coordinate their various activities under the professional guidance of the clinical director.

The chiefs of the various services in each hospital are also appointed by the association's board of directors and are responsible to the individual chiefs of clinical services for the organization and administration of the service to which they are appointed. Where appropriate, the chief of a service in a central hospital is responsible for policies in respect to his specialty in all affiliated institutions. The chiefs of the various services in the base hospitals also serve the affiliated hospitals as consultants in their specialties.

A liaison committee, composed of the chief of clinical services, the administrator, and the president of the medical staff, has been established in each hospital to coordinate medical and administrative affairs. The individual administrators serve as chairmen of these committees.

A regional medical board has been established for each regional or central group of hospitals. The chiefs of clinical services in the base hospitals serve as chairmen of these boards. The remaining members of each board consist of the chiefs of clinical services in the affiliated institutions and five chiefs of services from the medical staffs of the hospitals in the region. Each board has the responsibility of coordinating medical services in its region and maintaining medical standards. These boards also appoint the medical staff standing and task committees in each hospital in their region.

The Committee on Medical Affairs serves as a medical advisory committee to the medical administrator and the clinical director on matters concerning medical practice, medical education, and clinical investigation. The clinical director serves as chairman and the remaining members consist of the medical administrator, the three chiefs of clinical services from the central hospitals, and two to four members of the medical staffs of all the hospitals.

The medical staffs of the individual hospitals are organized locally and elect their own officers. Physicians practicing in the area served by the hospitals are utilized to the fullest possible extent and any qualified physician may obtain hospital privileges. However, about ninety of the key specialist posts are filled by full-time, salaried physicians.

Trends. Since the Miners Memorial Hospital Association has basically met its own health needs, it is doubtful that these events will greatly increase its significance to the hospital industry in future years. Yet this association demonstrates the willingness of labor unions to assume the responsibility of providing medical and hospital care to their members and families. However, it seems clear that most unions establishing health insurance programs prefer to use existing hospital facilities rather than build one or more hospitals of their own.

Patterns of Hospital Ownership and Control

One of the more unusual and comprehensive of the many health insurance plans evolving in the United States in recent years is the plan developed by the Kaiser Foundation (formerly the Permanente Foundation) on the Pacific Coast.

Organizational Structure and Governing Authority. The Kaiser system embodies four major principles — prepayment, group medical practice, preventive medical care, and integrated hospitals and medical offices — and consists of the following separate but interrelated entities:

1. The Kaiser Foundation. The parent organization is the Kaiser Foundation, a charitable trust initiated by industrialist Henry J. Kaiser and created by the California Kaiser Company for various purposes, including the furnishing of medical, nursing, and hospital care, scientific research, and medical education. The foundation sponsors the Kaiser Foundation Health Plan and holds title to the various hospitals, clinics, and rehabilitation centers which it leases to the Kaiser Foundation Hospitals. A self-perpetuating board of seven trustees governs the foundation and forms policies for all the separate entities.

2. The Kaiser Foundation Health Plan. The health plan is a nonprofit trust which enrolls members, collects dues, and maintains records of eligibility. For a basic monthly dues payment plus occasional additional charges, the plan provides medical, surgical, and hospital care to all subscribers and their dependents. Membership in the plan may be on a group or individual basis. The health plan "purchases" hospital and medical care for its members by allocating a certain portion of its revenues to the Kaiser Foundation Hospitals and another portion to the Permanente Medical Groups. Approximately 5 per cent of its revenues are retained by the plan for administrative expenses. The plan is governed by a board of five trustees consisting of Kaiser attorneys and industrial executives from the various Kaiser enterprises.

3. The Permanente Medical Groups. Medical and surgical care is provided to members of the health plan by the Permanente Medical Groups. These are independent groups of physicians organized as partnerships who staff and medically manage the Kaiser Foundation Hospitals.

4. The Kaiser Foundation Hospitals. These hospitals are nonprofit corporations which lease the facilities they operate from the Kaiser Foundation.

History of Growth and Development. The health plan has been in existence since the late 1930s. The plan was first introduced to Kaiser's dam project workers and during World War II was expanded to include his shipyard, steel, and other employees. At the end of the war, the plan was made available to the general public in areas where Kaiser medical centers existed. During the past few years, fifty thousand new members have been enrolled annually and the present membership exceeds 575,000 persons.

In 1942 the Kaiser Foundation assumed control of an 80-bed, existing hospital in Oakland, California, and built another in Vancouver, Washington. At present the foundation owns twelve hospitals, thirty-seven clinics, and two rehabilitation centers. Additional facilities are under construction.

Measures of Significance. All twelve hospitals are general-acute institutions. In 1957 their combined capacity was approximately 2000 beds and they admitted an estimated 75,000 patients, or about 39 admissions per bed. The average daily census exceeded 1300 patients and the average occupancy rate was nearly 68 per cent.

The hospitals ranged in size from 30 to 409 beds and the average capacity was more than 160 beds.

Over 2800 persons were employed in the twelve hospitals during the year, or roughly 2.1 employees per patient.

One of the hospitals was located in Washington, one in Utah, and ten in California.

Ten hospitals were members of the American Hospital Association in 1957 and all twelve belonged to state or regional associations. In addition, all that were eligible were accredited by the Joint Commission on Accreditation of Hospitals.

Financial Data. From data reported to the American Hospital Association for 1957, it was estimated the twelve hospitals expended nearly $18 million during the year and the cost per patient day exceeded $35.00. The latter was considerably more than the cost per patient day in all nonprofit hospitals in the United States but was slightly less than that of the nonprofit hospitals in the State of California, in which all but two of the Kaiser institutions were located.

Estimated payroll expenses in the same year were over $8.5 million and the payroll component of total expenses was about 47 per cent.

The income of the Kaiser Foundation Hospitals derives primarily from two sources: (1) a proportionate share of the health plan's prepaid dues, and (2) a variable amount from nonmembers of the plan who are the private patients of Permanente physicians and private practitioners. The rates charged nonmember patients are comparable with average hospital rates in the area.

Total capital invested in the twelve hospitals was estimated at approximately $35 million in 1957, or around $18,000 per bed.

Capital funds for new construction and expansion are obtained primarily from private sources, including commercial banks and Kaiser industrial enterprises.

Educational Activities. The Kaiser Foundation believes a health insurance plan must, in addition to being economically sound, provide teaching and training to stimulate a high quality of patient care and research to contribute to the future.

Three hospitals were approved for residencies in 1957 by the American Medical Association and two were approved for rotating internships. None of the hospitals were affiliated with a medical school.

The Kaiser Foundation School of Nursing — a three-year, state approved, professional nursing school — was established in the hospital in Oakland, California, in 1947.

Other educational activities include an educational leave program which has been developed for all Permanente physicians and the annual publication of a medical bulletin narrating some of the important contributions Permanente physicians have made to the advancement of medical knowledge.

Administration. The operation of each hospital is in the hands of a nonmedical administrator who coordinates his functions with the hospital's medical director. Each administrator is responsible to one of three regional hospital directors, who in turn is responsible to the trustees of the Kaiser Foundation.

Medical Staff. As stated previously, partnerships of physicians, known as the Permanente Medical Groups, staff and medically manage the Kaiser Foundation Hospitals. To be eligible for a partnership, a physician must have served in the group for three years on a fixed-salary basis. The groups, by contract, receive a proportionate share of the health plan's revenues, and incomes of individual physicians compare favorably with those of private practitioners in the same area.

Private physicians are permitted associate privileges in Kaiser Foundation Hospitals upon application and on the approval of a Medical Credentials Committee.

Trends. The Kaiser system of providing for medical, surgical, and hospital care is becoming increasingly significant. This is evidenced by the continual increase in enrollment in the health plan and by the expansion and new construction of hospitals and other facilities.

THE SHRINERS HOSPITALS FOR CRIPPLED CHILDREN

The Shriners Hospitals for Crippled Children are a group of seventeen institutions — thirteen in the continental United States, two in Canada, and one each in Mexico and Hawaii — devoted to the rehabilitation of underprivileged, orthopedically handicapped children.

Organizational Structure and Governing Authority. The hospitals are owned and operated by a fraternal order, the Ancient Arabic Order of Nobles of the Mystic Shrine of North America, and have been incorporated in the State of Colorado under the name "Shriners Hospitals for Crippled Children."

A national Board of Trustees, elected by representatives of the various temples at annual meetings, is the policy-making body and is responsible for the over-all management of the hospitals.

Individual hospitals are operated and managed by a local group of Shriners, designated as the Board of Governors, who are elected to their positions by the Board of Trustees.

Admission Requirements. The following requirements must be met before an orthopedically handicapped child is admitted to a Shriners hospital: (1) the child must be under fourteen years of age and mentally normal; (2) the child's parents or guardian must be unable to pay for the necessary hospital and medical care; (3) in the opinion of the medical staff, there must be the possibility of either completely curing the child or of rehabilitation to physical and social self-sufficiency.

Admission application forms must be completed and signed by a Shriner who is in good standing in his temple. The child must be examined by a physician whose report, together with the child's birth certificate and three photographs, must accompany the application. The various Boards of Governors review each application subject to approval or rejection.

History of Growth and Development. Almost all of the hospitals were established during the 1920s. The first units were opened at Shreveport, Louisiana, and St. Louis, Missouri, in 1922. The first Shriners hospital outside the continental limits of the United States was established in 1923 in Honolulu, Hawaii. The most recent addition was the hospital in Los Angeles, California, opened in 1951.

Measures of Significance. The Shriners hospitals are all long-term, orthopedic institutions. In 1956 they had a combined capacity of 1040 beds and admitted over 4000 patients, or about four admissions per bed. The average daily census exceeded 1000 patients and the average occupancy rate was approximately 98 per cent. The latter figure was much higher than the average occupancy rate in all orthopedic hospitals in the United States during that year and probably reflects the charitable nature of the Shriners institutions.

The hospitals had an average capacity of just over 61 beds in 1956 and ranged in size from two 30-bed institutions in Honolulu, Hawaii, and Mexico City, Mexico, to the 120-bed hospital in St. Louis.

The thirteen hospitals in the United States are well dispersed; each of the nine geographic regions of the American Hospital Association contains at least one such institution. The West North Central region contains two Shriners hospitals and four are located in the Pacific region.

Approximately 1100 persons were employed in the seventeen hospitals in 1956, or slightly more than one employee per patient.

Also in 1956, all seventeen institutions held accreditation by the Joint Commission on Accreditation of Hospitals and all were members of the American Hospital Association. In addition, at least fourteen were members of state, provincial, or regional hospital associations.

Financial Data. Accurate financial data on the Shriners hospitals are not available. However, the total capital invested in the seventeen institutions in 1956 was estimated to exceed $20 million, or about $20,000 per bed.

Shriners hospitals are financed by (1) an annual assessment of five dollars on each member of the Shrine; (2) the sale of life memberships to Shriners at a cost of one hundred and fifty dollars; (3) the sale of sixty-dollar contributing memberships which can be purchased by any person, association, corporation, or club; (4) bequests, endowments, and donations; (5) Shrine circuses, football and baseball games, and other fund-raising events.

As one of the admission requirements stipulates that the applicant's parents or guardian must be unable to pay for the needed hospital and medical care, no operating or capital funds are derived from patient sources.

Educational Activities. Thirteen Shriners hospitals were approved for residencies by the American Medical Association in 1956 and two were affiliated with medical schools. None of the hospitals was approved for internships and none offered programs in nursing education.

Administration. All of the hospitals are administered by women who are registered nurses. Each administrator coordinates her activities with the medical director and is responsible to a national administrator who is a member of the Board of Trustees.

The local Boards of Governors appoint their own administrators. However, the national administrator usually submits for the board's consideration the names of several persons qualified for the position.

Medical Staff. The final responsibility for the medical management of the Shriners hospitals is vested in a Board of Surgeons, the members of which are appointed by the Board of Trustees. The Board of Surgeons selects a chief surgeon for each hospital who acts in the capacity of medical director. He appoints an assistant chief surgeon and the other medical staff members.

All medical specialties are represented on each staff. However, most,

146

if not all, staff members have their own private practices and none, including the chief surgeons and their assistants, devote full time to the particular hospitals with which they are associated. Several members of each staff — usually the chief surgeon, his assistant, and the pediatrician — receive a small salary. All other staff members serve without pay.

Trends. Although a hospital was added to the chain in 1951, construction of new facilities and expansion of existing hospitals are not being carried on to any great extent. However, some Shriners hospitals are beginning to purchase care from other community hospitals and indications are that this practice will increase in the future. Thus it appears the Shriners Hospitals for Crippled Children will continue to remain relatively constant in their significance to the entire hospital industry.

ADDENDUM

Osteopathic Hospitals

Osteopathy is defined in the 1956 edition of *Webster's New Collegiate Dictionary* as "a system of medical practice based on the theory that disease is due chiefly to mechanical derangement in tissues, placing emphasis on restoration of structural integrity by manipulation of the parts. The use of medicines, surgery, proper diet, psychotherapy and other measures are included in osteopathy."

Practitioners of this science are known as doctors of osteopathy (D.O.) and institutions wholly or predominantly staffed by such physicians are referred to as osteopathic hospitals.

Organizational Structure and Governing Authority. Osteopathic hospitals vary greatly in their ownership and control. A few are governmental institutions controlled by counties and municipalities; however, the vast majority are nongovernmental in character. Of the latter group, approximately one half are owned and operated by nonprofit associations or corporations and the remaining one half are proprietary or "profit" enterprises.

Direct operating responsibility of the osteopathic hospitals controlled by nonprofit associations or corporations is usually vested in a board of trustees or directors in a manner similar to that of most nonprofit, nongovernmental hospitals staffed by doctors of medicine. These governing boards are composed of both doctors of osteopathy and lay individuals.

Roughly 45 per cent of the proprietary osteopathic institutions are owned by individuals, 25 per cent by partnerships, and 30 per cent by profit corporations.

History of Growth and Development. The osteopathic profession was born as a reform movement in American medicine. Osteopathy was originally propounded in 1874 by Dr. Andrew Taylor Still, a practicing physician who had served as a surgeon in the Union Army during the Civil War.

The first osteopathic hospital was also a teaching institution. It was

Patterns of Hospital Ownership and Control

operated in conjunction with the first college of osteopathy, incorporated in Kirksville, Missouri, in 1892.

The growth of the osteopathic profession over the years has been followed by a similar growth in the number of osteopathic hospitals and beds. In 1956 there were over 12,000 osteopathic physicians and surgeons in the United States and nearly 400 osteopathic hospitals were scattered throughout the nation.

Measures of Significance. The 1957 *Directory of the American Osteopathic Hospital Association* listed 392 osteopathic hospitals, with a combined capacity of 11,717 beds. Some hospitals with dual staffs — memberships comprised of both doctors of medicine and doctors of osteopathy — are included in this figure and some are not. During 1956 these 392 institutions admitted an estimated 630,000 patients, or approximately 54 admissions per bed.

Most osteopathic hospitals are general-acute institutions; less than five per cent provide a specialized type of service. The hospitals are typically quite small; in 1956 their average capacity was under 30 beds and they ranged in size from two to 322 beds. During the same year, an estimated 19,000 persons were employed in osteopathic hospitals, or about two employees per patient.

Osteopathic hospitals are not eligible for listing in the American Hospital Association's annual directory and therefore do not qualify for accreditation by the Joint Commission on Accreditation of Hospitals. However, the Bureau of Hospitals of the American Osteopathic Association — the osteopathic counterpart of the American Medical Association — has a hospital inspection and registration service that is similar to the J.C.A.H. program in its methods and objectives. Ninety-two osteopathic hospitals in the United States met the required standards and were registered by the American Osteopathic Association for the period from July 1, 1956 to June 30, 1957.

An obvious correlation exists between the number of osteopathic hospitals in a particular state, the number of osteopaths practicing in the state, and the degree of freedom allowed doctors of osteopathy by the state legislature. Thus there are usually more osteopathic institutions in states that allow osteopaths greater flexibility in their practice.

In 1956 nearly 61 per cent of the osteopathic hospitals were congregated in five states — Texas, Missouri, California, Michigan, and Oklahoma — and 67 per cent were located west of the Mississippi River. There were no osteopathic hospitals in Alabama, Arkansas, Connecticut, Idaho, Louisiana, Maryland, Mississippi, Montana, Nevada, New Hampshire, North Carolina, North Dakota, South Carolina, Utah, Vermont, and Virginia.

Financial Data. In 1956 the total operating expenditures of osteopathic hospitals were estimated at more than $70 million, or roughly $35.00 per patient day. Annual payroll expenses were estimated to be over $39 million, or nearly 55 per cent of the total amount expended.

Operating income is primarily derived from fees received from patients and third parties for services rendered. In some of the hospitals, the osteopaths on the staff pay a fee for each patient they admit.

The capital investment in land, equipment, and buildings in 1956 was estimated at $80 million, or approximately $6900 per bed.

In the past, osteopathic institutions found it difficult to raise money for construction or expansion through normal channels, and the osteopaths themselves were the primary source of capital funds. Today, although the bulk of the financing still comes from within the profession and from private sources, osteopathic hospitals are eligible to receive federal funds under the Hill-Burton Act, and new and expanded facilities are also being financed by the sale of bonds, by community fund-raising drives, and similar methods.

Educational Activities. Osteopathic hospitals are staffed by physicians and surgeons who are graduates of the six accredited osteopathic colleges in the country. Each college is a private, nonprofit institution requiring a minimum of three years of preprofessional education to gain admission. All osteopathic colleges require a training period of four years, or five thousand hours of academic work. Upon receiving the Doctor of Osteopathy (D.O.) degree, graduates serve a twelve-month internship in an osteopathic hospital approved by the American Osteopathic Association. Certification in a specialty field requires five additional years of training, including a residency and supervised study. All specialty fields of medicine are available.

Forty-four osteopathic hospitals were approved by the American Osteopathic Association for residency training and eighty-eight for internships in 1956. In addition, at least one osteopathic institution — the Philadelphia College of Osteopathy — operated a professional nursing school during the year.

Administration. Many osteopathic hospitals, particularly the smaller institutions, are both owned and administered by doctors of osteopathy. The remaining osteopathic hospitals are administered by nonmedical individuals in a manner similar to that employed in most other voluntary, nonprofit hospitals. A significant number of the osteopathic institutions in the latter group are managed by registered nurses.

Medical Staff. The staffs in most osteopathic hospitals have too small a membership to be organized in any formal manner. However, the staffs are usually divided by clinical services when the membership is of sufficient size to warrant such an organizational structure.

The American Osteopathic Hospital Association. The American Osteopathic Hospital Association is a national service organization for osteopathic hospitals and is very similar to the American Hospital Association in its program and organizational structure. Among other things, it holds an annual convention, sponsors institutes and a nursing scholarship program, maintains a library, provides consultation to member hospitals, and publishes a weekly newsletter, a bimonthly magazine, and an annual directory. The main office is in Davenport, Iowa.

Any hospital having one or more doctors of osteopathy on its staff which meets the following requirements is eligible for membership.

1. The hospital's staff members are to be members of their local, state, and national professional associations.

2. The hospital must have facilities and personnel to provide accredited care for inpatients on a twenty-four-hour per day basis. It must meet local and state health department requirements for a general and/or obstetrical hospital.

3. The hospital must maintain complete patient records.

4. The professional care of patients must be of such standard that the health and welfare of the patient will be protected.

5. All hospitals limiting care to specialties shall be identified as such.

Approximately 65 per cent of the osteopathic hospitals were members of the national association in 1956. In addition, state osteopathic hospital associations have been organized in California, Florida, Iowa, Kansas, Maine, Michigan, Missouri, New Mexico, Ohio, Oklahoma, Pennsylvania, Texas, and Washington.

Trends. The number of osteopathic hospitals and osteopathic beds in the United States has increased significantly over the years. In 1956 a survey of 265 osteopathic institutions indicated that forty-eight hospitals would have an additional 1306 beds ready for occupancy by the end of 1957, an 11 per cent increase in the total number of osteopathic beds in one year.

At this point it is realistic to assume that osteopathic hospitals will continue to grow and expand at approximately the same rate as in the past. However, their real future seems to depend on (1) the degree to which osteopathy and osteopaths are recognized by national, state, and local medical societies and the effect this recognition has on the activities of osteopaths; (2) the degree to which osteopathy and osteopaths are accepted by the population to be served; and (3) the degree to which restrictions on the practice of osteopathy are relaxed by the licensing agencies in the various states.

Eventually the basic differences will be eliminated and the two medical groups will become one, with some of these hospitals assuming the responsibilities of the usual community hospital.

154

Acknowledgments

The authors are deeply indebted to everyone who generously contributed information and advice on various aspects of the study, and especially wish to thank the people listed below. The titles following the names indicate the position held by each person when consulted, and may no longer be current.

C. L. ANDERSON, Commander, MSC, USN, Executive Assistant to Inspector General, Medical Bureau of Medicine and Surgery, Department of the Navy, Washington, D.C.

JEROME BIETER, Staff Consultant, James A. Hamilton Associates, Minneapolis, Minnesota.

B. E. BRADLEY, Rear Admiral, MC, USN, Acting Surgeon General, Bureau of Medicine and Surgery, Department of the Navy, Washington, D.C.

FRANK B. BREWER, M.D., Assistant Chief Medical Director for Operations, Department of Medicine and Surgery, Veterans Administration, Washington, D.C.

FRANK R. BRIGGS, Administrator, Abbott Hospital, Minneapolis, Minnesota.

ROBERT P. CHAPMAN, Executive Secretary, American Osteopathic Hospital Association, Davenport, Iowa.

JOHN BOYD COATES, JR., Colonel, MC, Director, The Historical Unit, United States Army Medical Service, Washington, D.C.

JOHN K. CULLEN, Brigadier General, MC, Director of Plans and Hospitalization, Office of the Surgeon General, Department of the Air Force, Washington, D.C.

ROBERT DERZON, Administrative Assistant, University Hospital, Bellevue Medical Center, New York, New York.

CLYDE F. DIDDLE, Director of Public Relations, Northern Region, Kaiser Foundation Hospitals, Oakland, California.

EDWARD J. FITZGERALD, Division of Hospitals, Public Health Service, Department of Health, Education, and Welfare, Washington, D.C.

F. P. GILMORE, Rear Admiral, MC, USN, Assistant Chief for Planning and Logistics, Bureau of Medicine and Surgery, Department of the Navy, Washington, D.C.

Patterns of Hospital Ownership and Control

O. F. GORIUP, Colonel, MSC, Executive Officer, The Historical Unit, United States Army Medical Service, Washington, D.C.

OREN GOVIER, Staff Consultant, James A. Hamilton Associates, Minneapolis, Minnesota.

OWEN HATLEY, Assistant Administrator, Charles T. Miller Hospital, St. Paul, Minnesota.

S. B. HAYS, M.D., Major General, The Surgeon General, Department of the Army, Washington, D.C.

V. M. HOGE, M.D., Assistant Surgeon General, Chief, Division of Hospital and Medical Facilities, Public Health Service, Department of Health, Education, and Welfare, Washington, D.C.

JOHN R. JEFFRIES, Assistant Administrator, Dr. W. H. Groves Latter-Day Saints Hospital, Salt Lake City, Utah.

CHARLES D. JENKINS, JR., Assistant Administrator, Memorial Medical Center, Williamson, West Virginia.

A. DOUGLAS KINCAID, JR., Staff Consultant, James A. Hamilton Associates, Minneapolis, Minnesota.

M. R. KNEIFL, Executive Secretary, Catholic Hospital Association of the United States and Canada, St. Louis, Missouri.

JOHN PARK LEE, Executive Secretary, National Presbyterian Health and Welfare Association, United Presbyterian Church in the U.S.A., New York, New York.

EDITH LENTZ, Director of Research, Course in Hospital Administration, School of Public Health, University of Minnesota, Minneapolis, Minnesota.

EDWARD LYNN, Assistant Administrator, Abbott Hospital, Minneapolis, Minnesota.

SISTER MARY MADONNA, Outpatient Clinic Director, St. Mary's Hospital, Minneapolis, Minnesota.

OSGOODE H. McDONALD, Secretary, American Baptist Home Mission Societies, New York, New York.

FRED A. McNAMARA, Assistant Division Chief, Hospital Programs, Hospital Division, Bureau of the Budget, Washington, D.C.

WILLIAM S. MIDDLETON, M.D., Chief Medical Director, Department of Medicine and Surgery, Veterans Administration, Washington, D.C.

ROBERT MORRIS, Social Planning Consultant, Council of Jewish Federations and Welfare Funds, Inc., New York, New York.

JOHN NEWDORP, M.D., Medical Administrator, Miners Memorial Hospital Association, Washington, D.C.

DAVID ODELL, Administrator, John Wesley County Hospital, Los Angeles, California.

OLIN E. OESCHGER, General Secretary, Board of Hospitals and Homes of the Methodist Church, Chicago, Illinois.

D. C. OGLE, M.D., Major General, The Surgeon General, Department of the Air Force, Washington, D.C.

TELMER PETERSON, President, Northern Pacific Beneficial Association, St. Paul, Minnesota.

Acknowledgments

CARL R. PLACK, Secretary, Lutheran Hospital Association, Washington, D.C.

CARL N. PLATOU, Administrator, Fairview Hospital, Minneapolis, Minnesota.

WAYNE C. ROHRER, Assistant Professor, Department of Sociology, University of Maryland, College Park, Maryland.

GEORGE M. SAUNDERS, Secretary, Board of Trustees, Shriners Hospitals for Crippled Children, Chicago, Illinois.

DAYTON SHIELDS, Administrator, Kaiser Foundation Hospital, San Francisco, California.

JAMES W. STEPHAN, Professor and Assistant Director, Course in Hospital Administration, School of Public Health, University of Minnesota, Minneapolis, Minnesota.

ROBERT E. VAN GOOR, General Manager, Group Health Federation of America, Chicago, Illinois.

CORINNE L. VOIGHT, Director, Shriners Hospital for Crippled Children, Minneapolis, Minnesota.

JERRY VOORHIS, Executive Secretary, Group Health Federation of America, Chicago, Illinois.

WILLIAM WALLACE, Administrator, Charles T. Miller Hospital, St. Paul, Minnesota.

CLARENCE E. WONNACOTT, Administrator, Dr. W. H. Groves Latter-Day Saints Hospital, Salt Lake City, Utah.

RAY WOODHAM, Administrator, Presbyterian Hospital Center, Albuquerque, New Mexico.

HAROLD K. WRIGHT, Director of Institutional Services, Board of Hospitals and Homes of the Methodist Church, Chicago, Illinois.

HELEN YAST, Librarian, Bacon Library, Chicago, Illinois.

LINUS A. ZINK, M.D., Deputy Director for Operations, Department of Medicine and Surgery, Veterans Administration, Washington, D.C.

BIBLIOGRAPHY

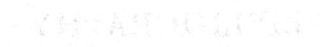

Bibliography

Books

American Medical Association. *Voluntary Prepayment Medical Care Plans.* Chicago: Office of the Association, 1950. 137pp.

Bachmeyer, Arthur C., and Gerhard Hartman. *Hospitals in Modern Society.* New York: The Commonwealth Fund, 1943. 768pp.

————. *Hospital Trends and Developments 1940–1946.* New York: The Commonwealth Fund, 1948. 819pp.

Cavins, Harold M. *National Health Agencies.* Washington, D.C.: Public Affairs Press, 1945. 251pp.

Commission on Hospital Care. *Hospital Care in the United States.* New York: The Commonwealth Fund, 1947. 631pp.

Commission on University Education in Hospital Administration. *University Education for Administration in Hospitals.* Washington, D.C.: American Council on Education, 1954. 199pp.

Corwin, E. H. L. *The American Hospital.* New York: The Commonwealth Fund, 1946. 226pp.

Faxon, Nathaniel W., Editor. *The Hospital In Contemporary Life.* Cambridge: Harvard University Press, 1949. 288pp.

Ginzberg, Eli. *A Pattern of Hospital Care.* New York: Columbia University Press, 1949. 368pp.

Gunn, Selskar M., and Philip S. Platt. *Voluntary Health Agencies.* New York: Ronald, 1945. 364pp.

Hiscock, Ira V. *Community Health Organization.* New York: The Commonwealth Fund, 1939. 318pp.

Mustard, Harry S. *Government in Public Health.* New York: The Commonwealth Fund, 1945. 219pp.

Rorem, Rufus C. *The Public's Investment in Hospitals.* Chicago: University of Chicago, 1930. 251pp.

Rosenfeld, Leonard S., and Henry B. Makover. *The Rochester Regional Hospital Council.* New York: The Commonwealth Fund and Harvard University Press, 1956. 204pp.

Sloan, Raymond P. *This Hospital Business of Ours.* New York: Putnam, 1952. 331pp.

Bulletins and Pamphlets

Administrator of Veterans Affairs. *Annual Report* (for the year ended June 30, 1956). Washington, D.C.: Government Printing Office, 1957. 347pp.

American Hospital Association. *Blue Cross Approval Program.* Chicago: Office of the Association, 1951. 19pp.

————. *The Blue Cross Concept.* Chicago: Office of the Association, 1948. 10pp.

————. *The Board's Control of Hospital Medical Care.* (Adapted from *Trustee, the Journal for Hospital Governing Boards.*) Chicago: Office of the Association, 1949 and 1950. 47pp.

————. *Federal Hospital Planning with Particular Reference to Care for Veterans.* Chicago: Office of the Association, 1947. 19pp.

————. *Veterans' Hospitalization Planning.* Chicago: Office of the Association, September 1950. 54pp.

American Osteopathic Hospital Association. *A.O.H.A. Directory for 1957.* Davenport, Iowa: Office of the Association, 1957. 104pp.

————. *A.O.H.A. Membership.* Davenport, Iowa: Office of the Association, 1956.

————. *Code of Regulations* (as revised Oct. 31, 1956). Davenport, Iowa: Office of the Association, 8pp.

————. *Directory of Intern Training Hospitals.* Davenport, Iowa: Office of the Association, June 1957. 47pp.

————. *The Growth of Osteopathic Hospitals.* Davenport, Iowa: Office of the Association, 1957. 16pp.

————. *Hospitals, Whose Responsibility?* Chicago: Office of the Association, January 1956. 18pp.

Anderson, Dewey. *Health Service is a Basic Right of All People.* Washington, D.C.: Public Affairs Institute, n.d. 70pp.

Board of Hospitals and Homes of the Methodist Church. *Answers for Ages.* Chicago: Office of the Board, n.d.

————. *Are We Doing Enough?* Chicago: Office of the Board, 1953.

————. *Blueprint for the Future.* Chicago: Office of the Board, 1957.

————. *Board of Hospitals and Homes of the Methodist Church.* Chicago: Office of the Board, n.d. 12pp.

————. *Institutions Affiliated with the Board of Hospitals and Homes of the Methodist Church — 1955–1957.* Chicago: Office of the Board.

————. *Methodism Speaks on Human Welfare Through Hospitals and Homes.* Chicago: Office of the Board, 1957.

————. *Methodist Philanthropies and Services in Hospitals and Homes for Children, Young Men, Young Women, the Aged, the Needy.* Chicago: Office of the Board, n.d.

————. *The Most Powerful Force in the World.* Chicago: Office of the Board, 1954.

————. *Prescription for Methodist Philanthropy.* Chicago: Office of the Board, n.d.

————. *Standards for Institutions Affiliated with the Board of Hospitals and Homes of the Methodist Church.* Chicago: Office of the Board, n.d.

Commission on Financing of Hospital Care. *Financing Hospital Care in the United States.* (Recommendations by the Commission.) New York: Blakiston, January 1954. 56pp.

Community Hospital Clinic. *Doctor Bills and Hospital Bills.* Elk City, Oklahoma: Office of the Clinic, n.d. 4pp.

Council of Jewish Federations and Welfare Funds. *The Council's First Quarter Century in the Service of the Jewish Communities.* Toronto: Office of the Council, November 1956. 10pp.

————. *Directory of Jewish Health & Welfare Agencies.* New York: Office of the Council, 1957. 42pp.

————. *The Jewish Hospital — Today and Tomorrow.* New York: Office of the Council, n.d. 27pp.

————. *Your Council's 1957 Budget & Dues Schedule.* New York: Office of the Council, 1957. 6pp.

Department of the Air Force. *Administration Manual of the U.S. Air Force. Medical Treatment Facilities* (Air Force Manual 160–20). Washington, D.C.: Government Printing Office, June 1956. 344pp.

————. *Appointment of Officers in the U.S. Air Force or as Reserves of the Air Force* (Air Force Manual A.M. 36–5). Washington, D.C.: Government Printing Office, July 1958. 48pp.

————. Office of the Surgeon General. *First Annual Report of the U.S.A.F. Medical Service* (for the period July 1, 1949 through June 30, 1952). Washington, D.C.: Government Printing Office, n.d. 287pp.

————. *Second Annual Report of the U.S.A.F. Medical Service* (for the period July 1,

1952 through June 30, 1954). Washington, D.C.: Government Printing Office, 1954. 401pp.

———. *Third Annual Report of the U.S.A.F. Medical Service* (for the period July 1, 1954 through June 30, 1955). Washington, D.C.: Government Printing Office, 1955. 473pp.

———. *Fourth Annual Report of the U.S.A.F. Medical Service* (for the period July 1, 1955 through June 30, 1956). Washington, D.C.: Government Printing Office, 1956. 621pp.

Department of the Army Medical Service. *Organization of Class I United States Army Hospitals* (Army Regulation No. 40-22). Washington, D.C.: Government Printing Office, April 1955. 27pp.

———. *Persons Eligible to Receive Medical Care at Army Medical Treatment Facilities* (Army Regulation 40-108). Washington, D.C.: Government Printing Office, December 1956. 25pp.

Department of the Army. Office of the Surgeon General. *Annual Report of the Surgeon General, Medical Statistics of the United States Army.* (Calendar Year of 1954.) Washington, D.C.: Government Printing Office, 1956. 344pp.

———. *List of Federal Medical Facilities in Continental United States.* Washington, D.C.: Government Printing Office, June 1957.

———. *Organization of the Office of the Surgeon General.* Washington, D.C.: Government Printing Office, July 1954. 118pp.

———. *Organization of the Office of the Surgeon General.* Washington, D.C.: Government Printing Office, January 1955. 7pp.

———. *Organization of the United States Army Hospitals Designated as Class III Installations or Major Class II Activities.* Washington, D.C.: Government Printing Office, February 1956. 50pp.

Departments of the Army, the Navy, and the Air Force, and United States Public Health Service. *Dependents' Medical Care.* Washington, D.C.: Government Printing Office, November 1956. 29pp.

Department of the Navy. Bureau of Medicine and Surgery. *M.D.–U.S.N.* Washington, D.C.: Government Printing Office, n.d. 32pp.

Emerson, Haven, Editor. *Administrative Medicine.* New York: Thomas Nelson, 1951. 1007pp.

Farmers Union Hospital Association. *Constitution and By-Laws.* Elk City, Oklahoma, September 1939. 15pp.

Freeman, Lucy. *It's Your Hospital and Your Life* (Public Affairs Pamphlet No. 187). New York: Public Affairs Committee, 1952. 32pp.

Hansen, Horace R. *Special Acts Affecting Prepayment Medical Care Plans.* Chicago: Cooperative Health Federation of America, 1956. 9pp.

Health Insurance Plan of Greater New York. *Health Insurance Plan Statistics Report for 1955.* New York: Office of the Association, 1956. 16pp.

Hospital Council of Greater New York. *Hospitals and Related Facilities in New York City.* New York: Office of the Council, 1955. 8pp.

Johnston, Helen L. *Rural Health Cooperatives.* Washington, D.C.: U.S. Department of Agriculture, Farm Credit Administration and U.S. Public Health Service, Federal Security Agency, June 1950. 93pp.

Lewis, Russel K. *How to Organize a Health Cooperative.* St. Paul: Health Center Services Commission, 1948.

Los Angeles County, California. *Los Angeles County Department of Charities.* Los Angeles: Office of the County, 1954. 48pp.

———. Civil Service Commission. *Meet the County. A Handbook for County Employees.* Los Angeles: Office of the County, April 1955. 35pp.

Lutheran Hospital Association of America. *Proceedings of the Seventh Annual Meeting* (September 10, 1955). Chicago, n.d. 46pp.

Lutheran Hospitals and Homes Society. *Bringing the Miracle of Modern Medicine to the Rural West.* Fargo, N.D.: Office of the Society, 1950. 20pp.

Patterns of Hospital Ownership and Control

Miners Memorial Hospital Association. *Hospital and Medical Care Plan.* Washington, D.C.: Office of the Association, n.d. 9pp.

National Archives and Records Service. Federal Register Division. General Services Administration. *U.S. Government Organization Manual 1956–57.* Washington, D.C.: Government Printing Office, June 1956. 782pp.

National Lutheran Council. Division of Welfare. *1957 Directory of Lutheran Agencies and Institutions.* New York: Office of the Council, March 1957. 52pp.

Northern Pacific Beneficial Association. *Changes in Constitution & Bylaws Effected May 18, 1955.* 1955.

———. *Constitution and Bylaws* (amended May 21, 1953). St. Paul: Office of the Association, 1953. 23pp.

———. *Seventy-Fourth Annual Report of the Northern Pacific Beneficial Association* (for the year ended December 31, 1955). St. Paul: Office of the Association, May 1956. 31pp.

Presbyterian Church in the United States of America. *Eighth Annual Report. Recommendations and Directory of the Division of Welfare Agencies for the Year 1957.* (As received and approved by the General Assembly of the United Presbyterian Church in the U.S.A., Pittsburgh, Pennsylvania, June 2, 1958.) 32pp.

Shadid, Dr. M. *Co-op Hospital Catechism.* Walla Walla, Washington: Pacific Supply Co-op, 1946. 48pp.

Shriners Hospitals for Crippled Children. Board of Governors, Twin Cities Unit. *Shriners Hospital for Crippled Children.* Minneapolis: Shriners, n.d. 12pp.

United Hospital Fund of New York. *Financial and Statistical Information Relating to Member Hospitals for the United Hospital Fund of New York and Hospital Statistics for Greater New York for the Year 1954.* New York: Office of the Association, 1955. 44pp.

United Mine Workers of America Welfare and Retirement Fund. *The Dedication of the 10 Memorial Hospitals.* Washington, D.C.: Association Office, June 1956. 25pp.

———. *Dedication of the 3-State Network of 10 Memorial Hospitals.* Washington, D.C.: Office of the Association, n.d. 23pp.

———. *Report for the Year Ending June 30, 1955.* Washington, D.C.: Office of the Association, 1955. 33pp.

U.S. Public Health Service. *Facts About Indian Health.* Washington, D.C.: Government Printing Office, 1956. 8pp.

———. *Health Services for Indians* (from Annual Report, 1956). Washington, D.C.: Government Printing Office, 1956. 8pp.

———. *Medical Internship in the Public Health Service.* Washington, D.C.: Government Printing Office, June, 1957. 12pp.

———. *Physicians in the United States Public Health Service.* Washington, D.C.: Government Printing Office, 1955. 20pp.

———. *The Public Health Service Today.* Washington, D.C.: Government Printing Office, 1953. 28pp.

———. Federal Security Agency. *Adequate Financial Support for Hospital Maintenance and Operation* (Public Health Service Pamphlet No. 76). Washington, D.C.: Government Printing Office, 1951. 27pp.

United States Senate, 82nd Congress, Committee on Labor and Public Welfare. *Health Insurance Plans in the United States.* (Report 359, Part I) Washington, D.C.: Government Printing Office, May 28, 1951. 114pp.

———. *Health Insurance Plans in the United States.* (Report 359, Part II) Washington, D.C.: Government Printing Office, May 28, 1951. 197pp.

———. *Health Insurance Plans in the United States.* (Report 359, Part III) Washington, D.C.: Government Printing Office, May 28, 1951. 44pp.

Veterans Administration. *Opportunities for Physicians in the Department of Medicine and Surgery.* Washington, D.C.: Government Printing Office, July, 1957.

———. *Veterans Administration Organization Manual.* (Introduction, revised 12-12-55, and Part I, revised 12-22-55.)

Veterans Administration Information Service. *Federal Benefits Available to Veterans and*

Their Dependents (VA Fact Sheet IS–1). Washington, D.C.: Government Printing Office, October, 1956. 14pp.

———. *Functions and Purposes of Veterans Administration* (VA Fact Sheet IS–10). Washington, D.C.: Government Printing Office, March, 1950. 14pp.

Voorhis, Jerry, and Robert E. Van Goor. *The Cooperative Health Federation of America and its Member Plans* (2nd ed.). Chicago: Office of the Federation, March 1955. 35pp.

Wallace, Thomas F. *Some Things I Remember*. Minneapolis: The Abbott Hospital, December 1953. 16pp.

Watkins, Bishop W. T. *New Tools for an Ancient Task*. Chicago: Board of Hospitals and Homes of the Methodist Church, n.d. 15pp.

Wicke, Bishop Lloyd C. *The "So What" That Really Counts*. Chicago: Board of Hospitals and Homes of the Methodist Church, n.d. 16pp.

Periodicals

American Hospital Association. Administrators Guide Issue, *Hospitals*, Part 2, August 1, 1957.

American Osteopathic Hospital Association. *The Osteopathic Hospital*. Vol. 1, Numbers 4, 5, 6, and Vol. 2, No. 1. July 1957 through January 1958.

Esselstyn, Caldwell Blakeman. "Group Practice with Branch Centers in a Rural Community." *New England Journal of Medicine*. March 1953, pp.488–493.

Featherston, William M. "I'm for Co-op Medicine." *Medical Economics*. Vol. 31, March 1954, pp.146–151.

Fowler, Jan. "Henry Kaiser's Medical Plan. More Care for Less Money." *Look Magazine*. September 9, 1952, pp.72–75.

Garfield, Sidney R. "Health Plan Principles in the Kaiser Industries." *Journal of the American Medical Association*. Vol. 216, No. 6, October 1944, pp.337–339.

———. "Permanente Foundation." *Medical Bulletin*. Vol. 10, August 1952, pp.1–11.

Memorial Hospital Association of Kentucky. "A Hospital Chain 250 Miles Long." *Architectural Forum*. November, December 1953, January 1954.

"Old Hospitals." *Southern Hospitals*. Vol. 5, No. 9, September 1937, pp.4–8.

Pollack, Jack Harrison. "Are There Holes in Your Health Insurance?" *Today's Woman*. December 1953.

Ramson, John E. "The Beginnings of Hospitals in the United States." *Bulletin of the History of Medicine*. Vol. 18, No. 5, May 1943, pp.514–539.

Miscellaneous

Davis, Newton. "A World-Wide Survey of Church Hospitals." (Columbus, Ohio, December 1938.) Mimeographed information, 7pp.

Freeman, Orville L. "The Prepayment Principle in Health Economics." (Dedication Speech at Two Harbors, Minnesota, July 18, 1957.) Reproduced by the Group Health Federation of America. 11pp.

Geetter, I. S. "Historical Development of Hospitals Under Jewish Auspices." Philadelphia: Council of Jewish Federations and Welfare Funds, September 1957. 5pp. processed.

Groeschel, August. "The Municipal Hospital: 1952." Philadelphia: Pennsylvania Public Health Association, October 3, 1952.

Hinds, Stuart W. "Historical Development of the Hospital." Geneva: World Health Organization, June 18–23, 1956. 10pp. processed.

———. "The Origin of the Word 'Hospital.'" Geneva World Health Organization Convention, June 18–23, 1956. 3pp. processed.

Jenkins, C. D., Jr. "The Regional and Central Service Aspects of the Operation of the Miners Memorial Hospital Association, Inc." (Bound thesis for the degree of Master of Hospital Administration, School of Hospital Administration of the Medical College of Virginia.)

Kaplan, Hyman. "Values of the Jewish-Sponsored Hospital to the Jewish Community." San Francisco: Council of Jewish Federations & Welfare Funds, September 1953. 8pp. processed.

Latter-Day Saints Hospital. "Policies and Procedures." (Prepared for the staff of Latter-Day Saints Hospital, Salt Lake City, Utah.) Mimeographed.

Lee, Russel V. "A Medical Utopia." St. Paul: Group Health Mutual and Group Health Association, March 1954. 8pp. processed.

Memorial Hospital Association of Kentucky, Inc. "Rules and Regulations Governing Medical Affairs, and Medical Staff By-Laws & Rules & Regulations." Washington, D.C. June 1955.

Mott, F. D. "A Hospital Chain for Coal Miners and their Communities." (A mimeographed release under the auspices of the Memorial Hospital Association of Kentucky, Inc., Washington, D.C. April 1954.)

——. "A Regionalized Plan of Medical and Hospital Care." (In a paper for the Memorial Hospital Association of Kentucky, Inc., Washington, D.C. April 1955.)

National Presbyterian Health and Welfare Association. "Report of Special Hospital Study Committee." Mimeographed release. 12pp.

Rusk, Howard A. "Hospitals for Miners." *The New York Times*, June 3, 1956.

Slawson, Robert, Editor. "1957 Yearbook of Jewish Social Services." Council of Jewish Federations and Welfare Funds. 38pp.

United Presbyterian Church in the U.S.A. "Relationships of Presbyterian Hospitals and Nursing Homes to the United Presbyterian Church in the U.S.A." Mimeographed release. 4pp.

U.S. Army Medical Service Historical Unit. "Summary of Major Events and Problems July 1, 1956 through June 30, 1957." (Prepared for the Department of the Army, Office of the Surgeon General, Washington, D.C., 1957.) 594pp.

U.S. Public Health Service. Division of Indian Health. "Indian Health Activities." (Opening Statement by Commission of Appropriations for 1957.) Washington, D.C., 1957. 18pp. processed.

Veterans Administration Information Service. "History of Veterans Medicine." (Mimeographed release, Washington, D.C., April 23, 1956.)

——. "How the Veterans Administration Developed." (Mimeographed release, Washington, D.C., December 15, 1954.

Weinerman, E. Richard. "Essentials of a Successful Group Health Plan." Chicago: Cooperative Health Federation of America, July 6, 1951.

166

Made in the USA
Monee, IL
07 July 2026

56552257R00103